ARI

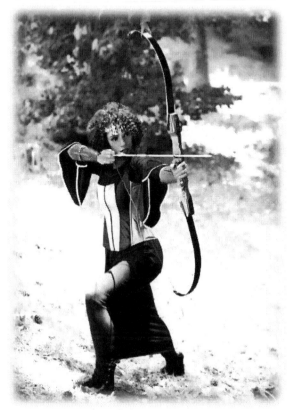

Alternative Medicine
Keys To Recovery From Opioid Addiction

By
DEVINA H. COLLIER
Biblical Naturopathic Practitioner
Certified Sclerologist, Iridologist
Certified Nutrition Consultant
Certified Natural Health Professional

DiVine Natural Solutions
A Private Healthcare Membership Association

Published by: Divine Natural Solutions.
Private Healthcare Membership Association.
P.O. Box 515 Flowery Branch, GA 30542 USA
DevinaHCollier.com
DivineNaturalSolutions.com
NaturalHealthEdu.com

All rights reserved. No part of this manual may be reproduced or transmitted in any form or by any means, electronically or mechanically, including photocopying, recording or by any information storage and retrieval system, without written permission from the author, except for the inclusion of brief quotations in a review.

Copyright © 2018 Divine Natural Solutions - Private Healthcare Membership Association.

ISBN-13: 978-0692157435. ISBN-10: 0692157433

Images By ReAnn Ring: Front, and Inside Cover.
Back Page Lion Image: © Can Stock Photo / Denisapro

All scripture quotations are from the Holy Bible, King James Version of the Bible and New King James Version of the Bible. Copyright © 1982 by Thomas Nelson, Inc., Publishers. All rights reserved.

Medical Disclaimer: Throughout history, dietary supplements and the right diet have been extremely helpful in helping the body to heal from sickness and disease. Devina H. Collier is not a physician or claiming to be a doctor. This book does not take the place of medical advice from a physician. This book is for educational and research purposes only. It is provided as a resource to bless you and teach you God's design for wholeness, health and wellness. An individual going through opiate withdrawal can have serious health complications. **Therefore, it is wise for individuals to speak with a healthcare provider first before taking dietary supplements or changing a diet.** Individuals should learn all they can about their unique biochemical needs before taking specific dietary supplements or foods to help them heal.

** If you have not done so already, by becoming a member of Divine Natural Solutions Private Healthcare Membership Association, you can receive natural health services via a private-client contract membership relationship that is not part of the public domain. For example, under the First and Fourteenth Amendments to the U.S. Constitution, we have 10 Liberty rights and guarantees; included is the right for an individual to contract, right to acquire useful knowledge, and right of freedom of association (freedom of speech, and freedom to join an association; organization, group or club without interference by the government). And freedom to worship God according to the dictates of the individual's own conscience. The U.S. Supreme Court has ruled overwhelmingly that U.S. Constitutional rights cannot be violated, noting that the State cannot interfere with private association activities unless the private members are being subjected to a clear danger of substantial evil that would shock a person's moral and common sense. Liberty rights were upheld in the cases of Meyers v. Nebraska, 262 U.S. 390; Board of Regents v. Roth, 408 U.S. 390; Flesher v. City of Signal Hill, 829 F.2d 1491; Estate of Marissa. Renee Imrie v. Golden Gate Bridge, Highway and Transportation District, 282 F. Supp. 2d 1145, Lawton v. Steele, 152 U.S. 133, Allgeyer v. Louisiana, 165 U.S. 578, Pierce, Governor of Oregon, et al. v. Society of the Sisters of the Holy Names of Jesus and Mary, 268 U.S. 510, and many other cases.

Dedication

To the Majesty, Great God, my King, the Physician, Jehovah Jireh, my Provider, Jesus Christ and His Holy Spirit – the Comforter. I Love You!

To my awesome husband of 23 years, Tirus, a United States Army and Coast Guard Veteran. I thank God for your prayers and support. Especially for keeping me healthy with mixing frozen mangos, blueberries, spinach, and raw okra smoothies every morning for me.

To the Reader, for having the courage to pick up this book, seeking God, allowing Him to take charge and breath life back into every cell, tissue, and organ in your body. Know this! There is more. God is your rear guard. Make ready! Aim! Command your day, and take it one day and one step at a time.

YES, you can bring your soul, mind, body and spirit into wellness. Put on the Whole Armor of God in health, knowledge, wisdom and power of the Holy Spirit of Jesus Christ.

** After you finish reading this book, please send me an email, letting me know how it helped, inspired or helped your recovery even better. Thank you, and God bless you and all of yours 😊

About Devina

Devina H. Collier is a Biblical Naturopathic Practitioner, Certified Sclerologist, Iridologist, Certified Nutrition Consultants and Certified Natural Health Professional. She is an author of several Biblically-Based Self-Healing Alternative Medicine Books. She is the founder of Divine Natural Solutions – a Private Healthcare Membership Association. She is a subject matter expert on natural health, alternative medicine (naturopathy – the study of natural medicine). She has an active private practice in Georgia, USA, and assists clients in-office, and online via Zoom.us, which is a Skype-like video conference platform. She practices biblical-based Iridology and Sclerology and does not practice any forms of New Age. Her faith is Pentecostal and bible believing. Her pastor is Jentezen Franklin from Free Chapel, Gainesville, GA. USA.

She is also the Alternative Medicine writer for The Christian View TV Talk Show's Online Magazine. They won 2 Awards for Best in Media in 2015 and 2016 and nominated for Rising in Community Excellence Awards in 2017 (RICEAwards). She has been on Atlanta Live TV 57 and spoke on radio and been interviewed live by women's ministries and is the host of Divine Women in Media and Ministries events.

The Whole Armor Of God

Ephesians 6:10-18: 10 Finally, my brethren, be strong in the Lord and in the power of His might. 11 Put on the whole armor of God, that you may be able to stand against the wiles of the devil. 12 For we do not wrestle against flesh and blood, but against principalities, against powers, against the rulers of the darkness of this age, against spiritual hosts of wickedness in the heavenly places. 13 Therefore take up the whole armor of God, that you may be able to withstand in the evil day, and having done all, to stand. 14 Stand therefore, having girded your waist with truth, having put on the breastplate of righteousness, 15 and having shod your feet with the preparation of the gospel of peace; 16 above all, taking the shield of faith with which, you will be able to quench all the fiery darts of the wicked one. 17 And take the helmet of salvation, and the sword of the Spirit, which is the word of God; 18 praying always with all prayer and supplication in the Spirit, being watchful to this end with all perseverance and supplication for all the saints.

Table of Contents

Dedication 3
About Devina 4
The Whole Armor Of God 5
Poems: 10
Worship At The Table and My Temple 10
Introduction 11
How Opioids Affected My Family 13
FDA Biggest Epidemic Crisis: Opioids 44
Alternative Medicine Evidence-Based Healing Foods 51
Allergies, Inflammation And Congestion 51
Circulation, Headaches And Migraines 53
Nausea And Vomiting 54
Indigestion, Flatulence And Constipation 57
Fatigue And Exhaustion 60
Muscle Pain And Soothing Support 62
Insomnia, Nervousness And Anxiety 65
Severe Anxiety, Stress, And Nerve Pain 68
Seizures / Epilepsy 71
Mood And Depression 73
Mental Confusion And Mental Fatigue 75
Fighting Infections 78
Emotional Balance For Courage 80
Emotional Balance For Grief 81
Emotional Balance For Anger 83

Emotional Balance For Stress 84
4 Elimination Systems of The Body 84
The Truth About Parasites And Recovery 89
20 Things That Weaken The Gut 94
50 Things That Support The Gut 95
Synthetic Sodium Nitrates (Salt) 102
Salt Choices 103
Hormone Disruptors 106
Trick Food vs Organic Food 112
Free Range vs. Cage Free Produce 122
Produce: Antibiotic, Hormones, Steroids 123
Grass-Fed Animals: Produce 125
Wild Caught Fish vs Farm Raised 126
Free Radicals vs. Super Antioxidants 127
12 Water Demands Of The Body 133
Types Of Drinking Water 134
Food Combining for Easier Digestion 141
Acidosis And Alkalosis 143
Acidic Foods 149
Alkaline Foods 150
Oral Health: Fighting Infections 151
Importance Of Natural Deodorant 154
Importance Of Natural Menstrual Products 155
BONUS DEVOTIONAL 156
Times Up Devil – Get Thee Behind Me! 157
Day 1: Know Your Real Enemy 157
Day 2: Don't Believe Lies Of The Enemy 161

Day 3: Illness: Satan's Advantage 164
Day 4: The Accuser 167
Day 5: Wrong Pride: Satan's Tactics 170
Matters Of The Heart: Breaking Strongholds. .. 173
Day 6: Unresolved Unforgiveness 173
Day 7: Unresolved Anger and Bitterness 177
Day 8: Unresolved Hurts 180
Day 9: Abandonment 183
Day 10: Soul, Emotional-Ties vs. Agape Love.... 185
The Heart Of God: Fruits Of The Spirit............ 189
Day 11: Love And Joy 189
Day 12: Peace And Reconciliation 191
Day 13: Kindness And Goodness 194
Day 14: Faithfulness 197
Day 15: Gentleness And Self-Control.............. 200
Renewal 203
Day 16: Restored And Healed..................... 203
Day 17: The Removal Of Sickness 206
Day 18: The Marvelous Body...................... 209
Day 19: Sustained And Strengthened 212
Day 20: Every Need 215
Mind, Will and Emotions 218
Day 21: Exhausted Soul 218
Day 22: Soul Care 221
Day 23: Isolation 224
Day 24: Walking In God's Presence 226
Day 25: Hope In God's Promises 229

Loving Yourself The Way God Loves You 232
Day 26: Help For Resentment 232
Day 27: Overcoming Rejection 235
Day 28: Overcoming Fear 238
Day 29: Temptation.. 241
Day 30: Idolatry... 244
Abiding In Christ.. 247
Day 31: Condemnation Or Conviction? 247
Day 32: What Your Heart Desires 250
Day 33: Faithful.. 253
Day 34: Born Again... 256
Day 35: True Identity...................................... 260
Motivational Gifts. Finding Your Calling 263
Day 36: Makeover 263
Day 37: Are You A Proclaimer?........................ 266
Day 38: Are You A Server?............................... 269
Day 39: Are You A Teacher? 272
Day 40: Are You An Exhorter? 275
Day 41: Are You A Giver? 278
Day 42: Are You An Administrator?................. 281
Day 43: Are You Compassionate?.................... 284
Day 44: Are You A Helper? 287
Day 45: Are You An Intercessor? 290
RESOURCES AND REFERENCES 293
80 Toxic Food Ingredients 293
U.S.A. Christian Drug Recovery Centers 296
How To Contact Devina?................................ 328

Special Thanks 329
Evidence-Based Clinical Trials: Alternative Medicine 330

Poems:
Worship At The Table and My Temple

By Poet, Angela Washington – Angel of Words!

Worship At The Table

From vitamin A, to vitamin B, I eat the foods, which strengthen me, veggies and water that removed waste, so I can be healthy, day to day. God placed the sun, to warm my skin. It blocked depression, and put joy in. Water helped detoxify impurities, because toxins congested me. Processed foods were not my friend, they damaged my organs. They aged my skin. Now, I know, what I must do, I'll eat to live, and worship you.

My Temple

Corinthians one and six tells me, my body is not mine. It is a temple made to serve. It is a worship sign. I can't eat anything. I can't stay up all night. I can't purge and binge. I can't eat what's in my sight. I have to be particular. I have to pick and choose. I may win the eating contest, but my body will surely lose.

Introduction

In this book you will learn God's way how to fight withdrawal symptoms with plant foods for a successful recovery from opioid addiction. Included in this manual is wellness living and a personal devotional to strengthen your faith and walk with Christ. When you have the strategies of Christ, you have the power to win.

In the beginning, God made the heavens, earth, day, night, seas, vegetation, stars, moon, sea creatures, birds, and animals. Lastly, the finished touch, He made something spectacular in His image. He made Adam and Eve and they were given an identity, purpose, and an assignment that included dominion over all the earth. Genesis 1: 1-31.

Incredibly, God formed Adam's body from the living nutrients of the dust (soil) and Adams organs became nutrients themselves. God then made those organs function and thrive by breathing life - a soul and spirit into Adams respiratory tract by way of his nostrils. This is why our words have power to speak life or death. Adam became a living soul and his body housed his soul and spirit. Genesis 2:7.

The right combination of balanced nutrients are keys for wellness because when nutrients are balance they have stronger unity to correct imbalances in the body. They are fuel - energy that our organs require to heal themselves and function. When organs are built up to become stronger then they can overcome withdrawal symptoms better.

Laboratory tests are done to evaluate blood, saliva, urine, and stool. Technicians look for illness and disease by the imbalance in nutrients in the specimen that came from a person's body. They also look for pathogen activities because some pathogens live off nutrients in human blood and those same pathogens can create malnutrition, and disease.

What is a nutrient? They are amino acids (protein), lipids, and carbohydrates, minerals, vitamins, bioflavonoids, polyphenols, and carotenoids. Essential elements are oxygen, carbon, hydrogen, nitrogen, calcium, phosphorus, potassium, sulfur, chloride, organic sodium, magnesium, silicon, iron, zinc, cobalt, manganese, copper, cobalt, iodine, selenium, molybdenum and chromium. Therefore, all these nutrients are needed in the correct balance to sustain and maintain a healthy body. Our spiritual food comes from the word of God, just like when God breathed life into Adam's nostrils and then Adam came alive. *"Man shall not live by bread alone, but by every word that proceeded out of the mouth of God."* Mathew 4:4.

How Opioids Affected My Family

I know that there are many families across this globe that have suffered the same, similar or worse things as my family did. That's why I do not mind telling the story of the circumstances in which I grew up because there is power in my testimony and it will help set others free.

My father's dad, Arthel, was a World War II United States Veteran. He had the wit of a genius, including the gift of carpentry. He and his wife, my grandmother, Genese LaVern moved from Texas to San Francisco, CA with their son, my father, James Arthel II and his sister. My grandparents had 9 children, which 7 were born in San Francisco.

It was in San Francisco where my parents met. My mother was gorgeous, tall, talented, smart, and well-spoken. I can see why my father was intrigued with her because she was a beauty. He was a strong man with big arms like Popeye's from the cartoon. His health was resilient too and I believe this was one of the reasons why my mom became intrigued with him. Unfortunately, she suffered with asthma and eczema but my father did not. Genese LaVern loved my mother, she wanted her as part of the family. I do believe God's hand played in this because Genese LaVern was a woman of faith and full of courage.

My mom truly loved my father and wanted to build a life with him. She had a heart of compassion and loved all babies. But my parents were still in high school and young. So, a future union was discussed by both my grandmothers, but it was Genese LaVern that asked my grandmother if her son could marry her daughter. My grandmother agreed to the union, and soon my parents traveled to Reno, Nevada and it was there they married.

Over a span of 8 years the babies came. I was born 2nd and the only girl-child my parents had. My mother gave me the middle name,

Renee, which is French and means "Born Again." Genese LaVern gave me my first name, Devina, which is derived from David, and is Latin, Scottish and Hebrew. It means "Divine, Beautiful, or Beloved." My mother's name, Betty, is Greek and means "Oath of God." Her middle name, Jean, is Hebrew and means "Gift from God." My grandmother's name, Genese is Greek and means "Genesis, Birth or Creation." My father's name, James is English, and means "The Eagle, Stone, or Bear." The mixed meaning of our names are "Birth, The Eagle, Oath of God, Gift from God, Born Again and Divine."

Road Blocks
When I turned 2 years old I developed chronic asthma, allergies and severe eczema which covered most of my body, including my scalp. Asthma was difficult to manage, especially when my mom smoked Kool's® cigarettes in the house which triggered asthma attacks in my lungs.

My father had God-given gifts - especially carpentry. He could fix many things like his father. But my father had problems. He didn't allow good role models to influence him, so He did what his peers were doing. He stayed away from church, drank alcohol, and was influenced by negative role models from T.V. Shows. He also decided he wanted 2 families instead of one, but this was not a joyous occasion for my mom.

He was absent most days in our lives, especially because of alcohol addiction. Alcohol is another central nervous system depressant, similar to opioids which slows down brain activity.

One day he got himself into trouble with the law, and that's when they told him to leave the city because he tried to force women into prostitution, including my mom, but she wouldn't do it. So, he became abusive towards her and abandoned us.

I was 3 years old just before he left the city. But he came to see me at my grandmother's house (my mother's mom). My grandmother was watching me while my mom was away. He asked if he could take me with him, but my grandmother sharply said "no." Then he kneeled, cried bitterly, hugged me, and said goodbye. I then watched him drive off in his car with his other family; my 2-half-brothers and their mom. I knew I wouldn't see him as much anymore, so I cried too. But to my surprise, I saw him a handful of times periodically after that, including my half-brothers and their mom. I wished to spend more time with them.

I spent one summer with him and I had fun. He gave me a classical piano and I tried to learn it by myself, but he soon sent me to day-camp with my brothers and cousins. My cousins were visiting for the summer as well. We really had a good time in Long Beach, California. My father kept a close eye on me and so did my brothers. I really bonded with my half-brothers because they took care of me and protected me. When day-camp was over, I watched my father manage an apartment complex and fix what needed to be fixed, including painting and plumbing, which he tried to teach me, but soon summer ended, and I went home.

When I was in 3rd Grade, my mom had a job, a car and a decent apartment in an upscale community in Daly City, CA. Considering the circumstances, she was doing well, and God blessed us. But when my father came to visit, things went downhill. Earlier on, he destroyed one of her cars. But she worked hard to get another one. It was a tan colored Cadillac, and we enjoyed it in our new community.

One evening he came to visit after a family funeral, but before he left the city he stopped by Daly City to see us. That day, he had been drinking. My mom let him in, and she looked radiant and happy. She was also glad to see him, so she cooked an early dinner and we sat down at the kitchen table to eat. It was quiet in the kitchen and we were told to stay in our chairs, but I got up after I heard my mom pleading with my father to stop. He trapped her in her room and hit her several times in her upper back with a long, thick, wooden object he broke off from her bed post.

I watched this attack and became hysterical and cried. My father saw me and told me to leave and shut the door, but I wouldn't do it. My mom heard me crying louder and turned and faced him and that's when the mighty hand of God stopped him from attacking her. I believe God triggered something in him, because the last time he saw me, I was 3 years old standing in the doorway of my grandmother's house waving goodbye to him as he drove away.

Witnessing that tragedy made me a stronger person. Especially because the only thing I could do was cry. But I have done a lot of healing and reflection since then, especially understanding who the real enemy was destroying the life of my mom and father. It was the evil one, the Prince of Darkness who Christ defeated on the cross at Calvary. That's why I choose to forgive my father, just as Christ forgave me.

My father left town again, and we could relax. So, we began enjoying our new apartment and the community again. We walked all over the hills and explored every inch of it. We were enjoying being together and settling in. My mom was an awesome mom and she was happy to be doing better.

Then another setback came within days. The Landlord cancelled my mom's lease. He said that we made too much noise and that the other tenants complained. So, my mom explained the situation to us. Then we packed up the Cadillac with our belongings. My mom had nice furniture, but she left it behind. Around the corner was a motel, so we moved there for a week while my mom went to work, and we went to school. Her job was across town at Presidio U.S. Army Military Base. Therefore, the Cadillac came in handy once again. I praise God for that!

Her coworkers and boss welcomed us on the base. My brothers and I went there a few times while my mom worked her shift. The base was a real treat for us to visit because it was perfect for kids to explore. I didn't understand all the historical landmarks, army tanks, or government buildings. But I was intrigued, nonetheless, especially because they let us play in the gym. Golden Gate Bridge was a five-minute walk from the base; 3-minutes if we ran. But my mom said no, so we just stayed put - but oh, how we loved the whole base. We have good memories, especially because they treated my mom well.

My mom's biggest concern was where we were going to live after the motel. Problems and concerns weighed heavy on her. She ran out of money just before God sent my grandmother to help us. My mom kept us together through thick and thin. She never separated us. That's why I thank God for her courage. My grandmother fed us and took us in too. She was a tremendous blessing.

Tender Place
We settled in my grandmother's house. We did not have beds, so we slept on the floor. My grandmother made us handmade pillows and

sewed our names into them from her sewing machine. She made custom quilts, so she gave us bedspreads to sleep on and it was sufficient. My mom was concerned about my growing bones lying on a hard floor, because she thought my bones would not grow correctly. So eventually she got a queen-sized bed and we all slept on it for a time.

During the transition into my grandmother's house, I had to change elementary schools. Mom's sweet voice was the first voice that woke me in the mornings before school. She whispered to me "RISE AND SHINE." ☺ Those words have a special meaning and tender place in my heart. Today, they help me remember her and all the good times and sacrifices she made. The hard times don't compare to those special words because those words bring God's light into every situation, past and present.

God never abandoned us. He gave us what we needed each day, and that was enough. We had food, clothes on our backs and a place to stay always.

My mom never left us at people's houses and she made sure we were clean, clothed and our hair combed. She was our nurse too! If one of us had a scrape on our knee, she would clean it and then bandage it. She took care of us like a mother should, and she did the best she could. These are the little things I appreciated about her. Especially for taking me to the hospital when I was sick. She and my grandmother helped me recover, and I was grateful for that.

Several times after school in junior high, my mom was there to walk me home. The kids teased me, yelled ugly things about the eczema on my skin. I tried to cover-up and hide my skin every day to prevent arguments and fights. Summer time was harder because it was hot, and hard to keep covered-up. But the kids still persisted, but I was not afraid to fight back, and when I did, I finished it and landed myself in detention after school.

When my mom came and got me out of detention, she'd wash my face, comb my hair and then take me up the street to Baskin-Robins® for ice cream and a soda pop. I loved that store, especially because my mom and I both had a sweet tooth.

My mom never blamed me for defending myself at school, nor did she punish me. She'd say, "I Didn't Raise Ugly Kids!" and that cheered and made me laugh. She had a funny sense of humor and loved to dance too, but drawing art was her finest hobby. She was a natural professional, not to mention having a keen eye for fashion as well. I liked to dance too, which really helped release stress. But there was a time when I lost the desire to dance after my mom's passing, but God gave me a new joy for dancing for him.

Opioids
My father attacked my mother every time he came to San Francisco. I believe the soreness she felt in her body from the blows to her organs drew her to opioids to numb the pain. Then that lead her to heroin addiction, which became a stronghold for the rest of her life.

She couldn't do much after that, and eventually stopped working at the Army base, but then went back the last 2 years of her life so we could collect her life insurance – which was not allot but it was sufficient. We used some of the life insurance to pay for her funeral, and Yes, it was a beautiful funeral indeed. For some reason, at the funeral, I would not cry, and did not cry for many years after that. But I know that through it all, my mom tried to do the right things for us, and she never stopped loving us. But heroin kept her in a cycle of relentless drug addiction.

Man can never fix his deep-rooted problems because that's for the mighty hand of God to fix. All we must do is allow Him to uproot it, no matter the pain. For example, pain last for a little while, while healing rises up from the ashes. When things get uprooted, there is a breaking or a tearing that takes place. Jesus reminds us to take the axe to the tree *"And even now the ax is laid to the root of the trees. Therefore every tree which does not bear good fruit is cut down and thrown into the fire."* - Matthew 3:10

All heroin did was masked the symptoms, but never healed the pain of the root problems. Heroin has miserable side effects. That's why I personally do not classify drugs as medicines because true medicines help strengthen the body with sustained nutrition for good health outcomes. They do not harm the mind, soul or body with deadly side effects.

My mom's availability became less. She stayed home and watched movies. But she did venture to the grocery and clothing stores, including other important places to buy necessary items or get services we needed. She couldn't do much more than that. My grandmother made sure we went to school because my mom faded out, sleeping a lot. We didn't understand or realize that she was high. She kept the addiction a secret for as long as she could. It truly felt like we had to raise ourselves, and frankly, we did at times. But God was still there blessing and protecting our family through it all because we were reaping the benefits from the prayers of our godly relatives before us, and my grandmother's daily prayers as well. It is a fact that prayer moves mountains for generations.

I began to move towards independence. I learned to catch the bus across town to my doctor's appointments. I found my way around the city by myself most of the time. It was a good thing, however that my mom and grandmother taught me how to catch the bus. But I did walk across town too. San Francisco was small enough for me to do that. I knew all the shortcuts through parks and over the hills which lead me back to my own neighborhood in an upscale community. I knew that God had been with me because I arrived at my destinations safely.

Gratefully, every couple of years my mom managed to buy me a bike, but I welcomed roller skates too. The bikes were useful getting me around the neighborhood, but it was hard to keep them from getting stolen. My baby brother had a skateboard and he was a professional on it. He was very smart because no one wanted to steal a skateboard. He used it on his Paper Route job, but then got more customers on his route, so then he purchased a bike with the money he saved. We were proud of him being so young and doing so well. He's still a hard-worker and is doing well today.

My grandmother encouraged me to take care of myself, work hard and get an education. My mom wanted the same things for me. I learned how to pray from watching my grandmother every night as she kneeled down to pray at her bedside. She and my aunt, Jeannette read the bible to me every day. They told me many times that Jehovah God loved me, which made a big difference in my life. Those days built my foundation in Christ. My mom's words reminded me to "RISE

AND SHINE." This helped me get up and look forward to new opportunities every day. God shined the light, and this light made me stand up and press on. I am grateful to my mom, grandmother and God for forcing me to think independently and differently.

The Purpose God Gave Me
I call the purpose, my calling in life; it's the calling God gave me. Without a doubt deep down in my heart, I knew God could heal every sickness and disease regardless the situation. In a hospital room, I watched Genese LaVern suffer severely from high blood pressure. The doctors said they couldn't do much more. I thought to myself, are you kidding me? Fix this! But this just ignited a fire in my spirit to help the sick to heal.

I simply did not want to see these fixable health problems go unanswered anymore. I was over being sick myself, but I didn't know how to heal myself. No one had the right answers, but the same answers with the same prescriptions and same expectations. Which to me wasn't a good enough answer. I knew my God could heal all sickness and disease. He is the one that created man, and He knew the keys to healing and recovery.

It's ironic, however, that I don't remember asking God to heal me. But I do remember asking Him to help me breathe when I couldn't. It wasn't until later in life after I got married that I asked Him to show me how to heal, and He did just that. Today, I wonder what my health would have been like if I asked Him to show me how to heal when I was a child or teenager.

Genese LaVern passed away from that high blood pressure. But now I understand her doctors did the best that they could with allopathic drugs. Therefore, I don't blame them, however, because we all need to be accountable for our own health and seek God for answers before seeking them from man. No doubt, God is the Great Physician. He is the true healer!

I was 12 years old when God did something special. He ignited a relentless hunger for His healing ministry. Genese LaVern's passing had an impact on me too. That's when I knew my calling was medical, health and healing. But I was born with this gift already, but God had to ignite it first - which really turned into a type of justice for me to see the sick healed, the right way – God's natural way.

I just didn't understand what to do about this calling God gave me. That's when I began a habit of walking through Glen Canyon Park after school to spend quiet time with God. It was there, I danced, and praised Him. I also climbed up the gymnasium roof so that I could fix my eyes on the whole forest to see more of God's creation. I walked the park's trails and analyzed plants, flowers, and trees. I spent hours looking, touching and smelling them. At the same time, asthma, allergies and eczema inflicted me and I had to use the asthma inhaler so I could breathe – but God was with me and I knew He was. I didn't know some of the plants I seen could heal me and others from sickness and diseases, including emotional stress.

When I turned 18 years old I enrolled myself in a private Medical Assisting School in downtown San Francisco. I took out a student loan of $5,000, and yes, I thought I was signing my life away. However, I knew I did the right thing because I needed to be in this field.

My mom and grandmother supported me with $2 - $5 in lunch money every day and a bus pass to get to school. I ate candy bars and other junk foods from the vending machines.

Those foods were toxic, but I didn't make the connection that they were keeping me sick. At home my diet was collard greens, beans, rice, boiled or fried chicken, pork chops, chicken and dumplings, hot dogs, spaghetti, spam, hamburgers, salami, pizza, hot and cold cereal, peanut butter and jelly sandwiches, cupcakes, cakes, pies, cookies, ice cream, soda pops, Kool-Aid® and other comfort foods. All was absent from the diet with what I actually needed to heal, except collard greens.

I started school right away. Some of the medical curriculum was challenging to understand, but medical terms were easy for me because the roots, suffixes and prefixes were in Latin. I grew up with Hispanic friends and learned some conversational Spanish from them. I also learned Spanish in high school. So, everything was right on time.

I found the cardiovascular system to be more complex than other organ systems, but it did not matter to me how long it took me to understand it, I would not quit. It amazed me how powerful organs were. For example, the detailed, intricate things they did to keep a man alive, even when his physical life was threatened. This fascinated me how God created the human body and how it's automatically programed to survive.

We had homework for several specialties. All the students helped one another get through homework assignments, plus we had teams. I remember this one dear student stayed after school to finish her clinical. She forgot to pour water inside the incubator machine we needed to grow bacterial cultures. The next day we came to class, we found the incubator had blown out thick, black smoke, but gratefully the incubator was not badly damaged. The white wall behind it was covered in black smoke. We all had a good belly laugh looking at this until we realized we could not pass our clinical without it. So, quick, fast and in a hurry, the wall got cleaned-up and the incubator thriving once again, and we all passed our clinical soon after that.

My First Volunteer Job
After several months of intense training, I graduated, but couldn't find a job. So, my grandmother told me to volunteer to gain experience first, so I did and landed a volunteer position in a nursing home as a nursing aide. The nurses on my shift were overworked, and I was

exhausted myself. After roughly 2 months, I did not want a career there, so I landed a different volunteering job at a hospital as a Phlebotomist in the outpatient laboratory at Presbyterian Hospital in San Francisco. I was so happy to volunteer at this historic hospital. I saw it as a whole new world with bigger opportunities.

It was hard to get this volunteer job at first. They told me "no" and refused to let me train on their patients. But I stayed around anyway and greeted the patients as they walked in for lab work. I was hoping that one of them would give me their arm to practice. I knew I could draw blood. Then, God moved mountains for me. The lab manger took me under her wings, and trained me whenever her supervisor was not around. I learned everything in a short period of time and became proficient. The lab manager appreciated me being there because it afforded her the ability to take needed breaks. I appreciated her sacrifices and I thanked God for answered prayer.

The hospital director noticed me and called me into his office. He handed me a Phlebotomy exam to see if I could pass it. I did pass it on the first try. He then gave me a written exam in which I had to write the answers on a chalk board in front of him. But, was I nervous? No, I was confident! After I passed it, he awarded me a Certificate of Achievement as Certified Phlebotomist with the hospital's stamp of approval. I walked out of there, held my head up high and had a dance in my spirit.

I thought, surely, I could get a paying job now. But there were no openings in the laboratory. So, I stopped volunteering after 3 months when God opened a door of employment across town. I landed my first full-time front and back office-medical assistant job in San Mateo. I was very happy to finally collect a paycheck, buy new clothes and eat what I wanted. I was able to save and buy a used car too - my "bucket" because it had maintenance issues and was on its last leg. Nonetheless, I was glad to have it and get to work in the mornings.

Now I was officially a grown up! I heard people say, you are not grown until you start paying your own bills. Well, I had those and payed my grandmother rent 😊 My mom said I was ungenerous because I would not buy her cigarettes. I remember trying to smoke cigarettes a few times as a teenager, and it nearly knocked me out and gave me a headache every time. So, I left that alone, quick, fast and in a hurry!

My Mom's Last Days
What lead to my mom's passing was that she unknowingly used a syringe infected with HIV from someone. She then developed AIDS from it and it eventually took her life. It was the last two years of her life was when she told us she had the virus.

Still, she tried to feel better and do better and received methadone to wean off heroin – but today, I understand that this was just as addictive because it was still an opioid. To no avail, she became very ill still and could not pick up her methadone anymore. She had no energy to catch the bus across town to get it. I remember driving her to the clinic to get it one time, but after that she didn't ask me anymore because I was working during the day. My mom had all these needs and my mind was somewhere else. Being so young, I didn't fully see or understand the urgency of the hour. I didn't realize her time was shorter than what I could see - she was not going to live long.

Then one day, my grandmother explained the severity of the situation, which finally got my full attention. She told us to prepare, stay close and do all we could to help. But my mom's declining health occurred quicker than I could imagine, and I could not keep up. Time ran out! All I could do was go to the grocery store, cook her meals, assist her to the restroom and sterilize the dishes and wash them for her. I learned about how the virus worked and how infection spreads, so I wasn't afraid to help my mom. But God gave my grandmother wisdom, and she wasn't afraid of the virus either.

My grandmother did everything. She managed my mom's care with tender loving patience and kindness. She was there full-time, day and night helping my mom. What an amazing Queen, she was for my mom. Came hell or high water, she never abandoned us.

God sent my mom a Hospice Care nurse to the house and she came every week day. We thanked God for the city of San Francisco for this incredible woman because my mom needed professional care. Her name was Ms. Thelma, and she helped during the day. We all appreciated her being there. My mom loved her because she went above and beyond with her care. She helped all of us and she became like an aunt to me and a friend to my grandmother. She gave us emotional support and tried to help us mend our family hurts too. She was a true gem from God! Ms. Thelma, if you are reading this, I want to tell you, thank you and bless your household!

The severity of symptoms my mom began to feel caused her great pain. She was in and out of the hospital because of complications. Eczema covered her body like never before. Her doctor was out of options and could not control it. But I knew a way to kill it immediately. So, I asked the nurse at the front desk for a roll of plastic Saran™ wrap. I then slipped plastic gloves on my hands and took my mom's prescription of Hydrocortisone cream and lathered her skin with it from neck to toe. I emptied two tubes. I then wrapped her body from neck to toe with the Saran™ wrap. She relaxed and finally went to sleep. The next day, I came to check her skin and saw the plastic wrap laying at her ankles as she stood at the restroom door about to take a shower. She smiled back at me, and kicked the plastic wrap off her ankles. I noticed the eczema was off her body and some of the dead skin from the eczema was stuck onto the plastic wrap. The eczema was choked to death and could not breath, and my mom's skin healed and was smooth like baby skin.

More so at home, the opioid withdrawal symptoms and virus was causing her great pain. She did not go through an opioid detox. She had little patience and yelled a lot. I didn't want to be in the same room at times, especially because her cigarette smoke triggered asthma attacks in me, and I struggled with that. I felt that she didn't care whether I could breathe or not, but I know this was furthest from the truth. My mom had an addiction and she was trying to cope with how it affected her. I wonder, if she realized how it affected the family, because for one thing I did not hear her talk about it. But one thing was for sure, she kept us together and we were a family - not in an odd way, but in a survival type of way.

Another time at the hospital, I wanted her to know how much I loved her. So, I told her, and apologized for giving her a hard time at times. I danced for her, and she watched me right there in her bed. Honestly, being uneducated about opioids at the time, at home, I didn't realize that my mom was experiencing withdrawal symptoms when she yelled at us. I just thought that she was angry. But now I understand that was furthest from the truth. Withdrawal symptoms are painful like the flu, and when people are hurting they're irritable and irrational.

The Last Day I Seen My Mom Alive
The day before she passed away, I met a pastor at a function. He told me the Lord's salvation and the sinner's prayer, and told me to say that to my mom. So, I went straight to the hospital where she was and quoted it to her. I asked her if she wanted to accept the Lord Jesus Christ as her Savior. She looked at me but could not speak. So, she cried instead. I had never seen her look like that before. Her face was like a baby with tears in its eyes. I said "mama, I know you can hear me. All you have to do is accept Jesus in your heart and He will save you." Then she tried to tell me something, but her pain was greater, so she continued to cry. That was the last night I had with my mom. She passed away in the middle of the night, which I did not expect it at all.

What I learned that quiet day, was that life is precious and none of us should take it for granted. We should be telling each other how much we love each other. We should be celebrating and helping one another do better.

Family is an inheritance from the Lord. Corrupt behavior is man's sin nature that's countered by divine nature.

My Father's Passing

My father was ill himself, but whatever other reasons, he did not call or check on us, nor did he come to my mom's funeral or burial ground. That doesn't mean, however, that he didn't mourn in his own way when he found out what happened. His liver hemorrhaged from alcohol damage. It was cirrhosis of the liver. He died on the same month, 1 year apart from my mom. My parents never divorced.

Some of the positive things I liked about my father was his laughter, hard-working ethic, gift of carpentry, talents and traits. I am especially grateful for inheriting his genes and the genes of his hard-working parents and their parents before them. God planned my destiny through their genes, and I won't complain because God's will still stands, and I am not a mistake. Jesus Christ is still on the throne.

Journey in Alternative Medicine

Apart from Jesus, the happiest day of my life was when I got married. Unfortunately, asthma, allergies and eczema became worse for me every year. I did not want my husband worrying and seeing me suffer like that all the time. The steroids and antihistamine drugs were expensive. I did not want to take them or buy them any longer. I was disheartened with going to my doctor's appointments every month - sometimes weekly. I wanted to save our money for other things, like a house, new car, clothes, and vacations.

I became exhausted with the cyclic routine of allopathic preventative medicine for my care because it was draining me, my health, budget, and not fixing my health problems. However, it did save my life many times. Nobody talked to me, however, about my diet to see if that was making me sick. It wasn't until my natural health studies, that I found my diet was a BIG factor why I was sick. I learned that I could heal if I changed my diet.

I simply wanted to enjoy my new life, so I asked God to heal me. But one thing came first. I needed the HELPER - the Spirit of the Lord. The Holy Spirit. The journey started when I went to Philadelphia, Pennsylvania to visit my mother-in-law for 2 months while my husband was working at sea. He was in the United States Coast Guard on patrol. My mother-in-law took me to her church every time the doors opened. The church was called "Apostolic House Hold of Faith." They were bible believing and working in all the gifts of the Holy Spirit. In other words, God presence was there. I never experienced anything like that before. People were sharing their testimonies how God delivered them out of difficult situations, and it was a beautiful thing to see.

I realized how thirsty I was for God. I did not know about the Holy Spirit. Growing up, I was taught the Jehovah's Witnesses religion, but I read from both the King James Holy Bible and their bible. But they had different views and did not believe the things I had seen or experienced in my mother-in-law's church. So, I decided to learn straight from the Holy Bible, the King James version. I also did a lot of research to find the truth. I discovered it took the apostles and disciples of Jesus Christ 1,500 years to complete the entire God inspired Holy Bible. It is highly organized and planned by the Father, Jesus Christ, Jehovah God. If God can give Adam in the garden instructions, Moses and Abraham instructions, then He can give anyone instructions.

Jesus Christ is the same today as He was yesterday. He was the one sending us help in both the good and bad times. Not only is He Lord, but the living Word and God all by Himself.

In the beginning was the Word, and the Word was with God, and the Word was God. The same was in the beginning with God. All things were made by him; and without him was not any thing made that was made. In him was life; and the life was the light of men. And the light shineth in darkness; and the darkness comprehended it not. John 1:1-5.

For unto us a child is born, unto us a son is given: and the government shall be upon his shoulder: and his name shall be called Wonderful, Counsellor, The mighty God, The everlasting Father, The Prince of Peace. Isiah 9:16.

In the basement of my mother-in-law's church, my husband and I were baptized together. 2-weeks later, I was Born Again and received the Holy Spirit with the evidence of speaking in tongues on December 12, 1996. My husband received the same soon thereafter.

And they were all filled with the Holy Ghost, and began to speak with other tongues, as the Spirit gave them utterance. Acts 2:4. And these signs shall follow them that believe; In my name shall they cast out devils; they shall speak with new tongues. Mark 16:17

So, I decided to step off the grid of allopathic medicine and go the way God lead me to go towards natural wellness. So, I enrolled in school full-time and received a natural health education. It cost thousands of dollars but was worth every penny. I excelled at that program and finished 3-years earlier, even though it was a 5-year program. How did I do it? God, massive focus, speed reading, good notes, and my medical background - especially anatomy and physiology. I have also studied at several other naturopathic training schools, and here I am today with several certifications, and an active practice.

I no longer suffer from chronic health issues, nor take pharmaceuticals to mask symptoms. I healed myself with dietary supplements, specific foods, and a healthy living strategy to keep my organs well. I am, however, still susceptible to asthma, eczema, and allergies, but thank God I am 90% better than I was.

FDA Biggest Epidemic Crisis: Opioids

Drug addiction has spread to all countries of the world, and the biggest crisis is in the United States. The data are more than alarming and the epidemic can freely be declared! But one truth remains, and that truth is quite simple - Every single drug is dangerous. Parents and guardians must not think that drug abuse is a phenomenon that does not concern them - that it's only a problem of others. No family is spared the possibility of one day entering that circle.

"The epidemic of opioid fatalities continues to deteriorate. The abuse of prescription drugs and the use of heroin and illegally produced fentanyl are interconnected and highly troubling problems," said Tom Freidan, the director of the CDC (Centers for Disease Control and Prevention), a federal agency in charge of public health. The World Health Organization (WHO) has estimated that worldwide that there are 15 million people addicted to illicit and prescription opioid drugs, and only 10% receive effective treatment even though there are treatment centers available. 69,000 deaths occur from overdoses yearly.

Source: CDC.gov
Chart: Drug Overdose Rate Increase By Highest to Lowest
www.cdc.gov/drugoverdose/data/statedeaths.html

STATE	2010 RATE	2016 RATE
West Virginia	28.9	52.0
Ohio	16.1	39.1
New Hampshire	11.8	39.0
District of Columbia	12.9	38.8
Pennsylvania	15.3	37.9
Kentucky	23.6	33.5
Maryland	11	33.2
Massachusetts	11	33.0
Delaware	16.6	30.8
Rhode Island	15.5	30.8
Maine	10.4	28.7
Connecticut	10.1	27.4
New Mexico	23.8	25.2
Tennessee	16.9	24.5
Michigan	13.9	24.4
Indiana	14.4	24.0
Florida	16.4	23.7
Missouri	17	23.6
New Jersey	9.8	23.2
Utah	16.9	22.4
Vermont	9.7	22.2
Louisiana	13.2	21.8
Nevada	20.7	21.7
Oklahoma	19.4	21.5
Arizona	17.5	20.3
North Carolina	11.4	19.7
Wisconsin	10.9	19.3
Illinois	10	18.9
South Carolina	14.6	18.1
New York	7.8	18.0
Wyoming	15	17.6
Alaska	11.6	16.8
Virginia	6.8	16.7
Colorado	12.7	16.6
Alabama	11.8	16.2

Armor of God

Idaho	11.8	15.2
Washington	13.1	14.5
Arkansas	12.5	14.0
Georgia	10.7	13.3
Hawaii	10.9	12.8
Minnesota	7.3	12.5
Mississippi	11.4	12.1
Oregon	12.9	11.9
Montana	12.9	11.7
California	10.6	11.2
Kansas	9.6	11.1
Iowa	8.6	10.6
North Dakota	3.4	10.6
Texas	9.6	10.1
South Dakota	6.3	8.4
Nebraska	6.7	6.4

Rates shown are the number of deaths per 100,000 population. Age-adjusted death rates were calculated by applying age-specific death rates to the 2000 U.S standard population age distribution.

THE OPIOID EPIDEMIC BY THE NUMBERS

IN 2016...

116
People died every day from opioid-related drug overdoses

11.5 m
People misused prescription opioids¹

42,249
People died from overdosing on opioids²

2.1 million
People had an opioid use disorder¹

948,000
People used heroin¹

170,000
People used heroin for the first time¹

2.1 million
People misused prescription opioids for the first time¹

17,087
Deaths attributed to overdosing on commonly prescribed opioids²

19,413
Deaths attributed to overdosing on synthetic opioids other than methadone²

15,469
Deaths attributed to overdosing on heroin²

504 billion
In economic costs³

Sources: ¹ 2016 National Survey on Drug Use and Health, ² Mortality in the United States, 2016 NCHS Data Brief No. 293, December 2017, ³ CEA Report: The underestimated cost of the opioid crisis, 2017

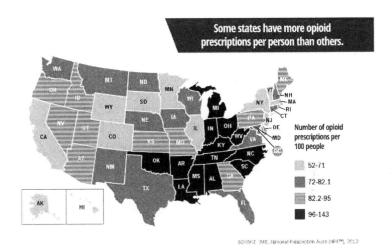

Source: www.cdc.gov/drugoverdose/data/prescribing.html

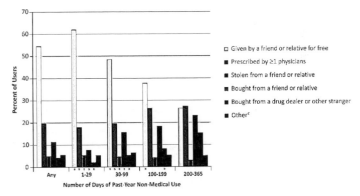

In addition to the fact that drugs are harmful to the physical health of a person, it is also harmful to his mental health.

Physical damages that have been reported with the use of opiates are hepatitis, HIV infection, damage to the bloodstream, stroke, heart attack (infarction), damage to the nasal mucosa and nasal cartilage, rapid heartbeat, dry mouth, severe dehydration, increase in body temperature, heatstroke, muscle spasms, brain damage, blurred vision, increased blood sugar, sweating, nausea, vomiting, and death due to heat shock or heart failure, and overdose.

Mental and Emotional damages that have been reported with opioid use are chronic depression and alienation, difficulties in thinking, reduction in memory and learning ability, loss of life interest and motivation, mood disorders, anxiety, disorientation, mental deterioration, psychosis, manic-depressive states, sleep disorder severe depression and anxiety, anorexia, reduced motivation or depressed mood that lasts for days, and suicidal ideas.

Armor of God

Graphic Sources (opioid side effects): WikiJournal of Medicine/Medical gallery of Dr. Mikael Häggström.

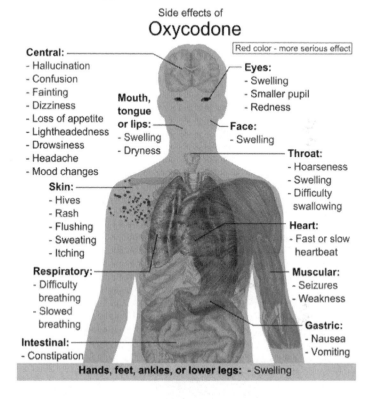

Armor of God

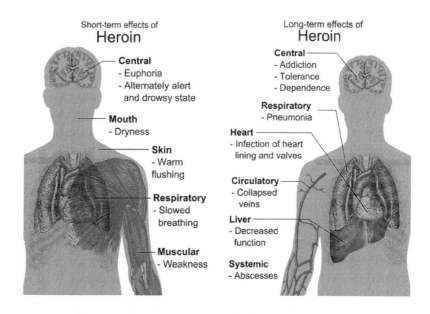

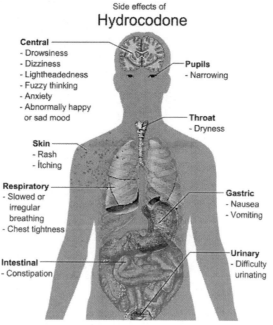

Alternative Medicine Evidence-Based Healing Foods

And as day was about to dawn, Paul implored them all to take food, saying, "Today is the fourteenth day you have waited and continued without food, and eaten nothing. Therefore I urge you to take nourishment, for this is for your survival, since not a hair will fall from the head of any of you."
Acts 27:34

Allergies, Inflammation And Congestion

Butterbur: It is an equatorial plant found mainly in Asia, Africa and some parts of Europe. Its extracts are mainly used in health problems like asthma, headaches, and allergies. A clinical trial conducted on humans has found that Butterbur is more effective in relief of the symptoms of rhinitis.[1]

Garlic: It has been popular for centuries. The bulb of the plant has well-known health benefits. It is especially known for its anti-inflammatory properties which makes it an effective herb for the relief of allergic rhinitis. Garlic helps with the reduction of inflammation. Trials on both animals and humans have proven garlic to be an effective treatment of allergies.[2]

Ginger: The gingerol extract in ginger reduces the production of substances which give rise to allergies and allergic rhinitis, according to clinical trials. The trials have shown a reduction in severity of sneezing and itchiness of the face as well.[3]

Spirulina: It is a blue green algae used to strengthen the immune system. Clinical trials on humans have shown that spirulina helps in reduction sneezing, nasal discharge, nasal congestion and itching.[4]

Moringa oleifera: It is a tropical and subtropical plant well known for its medicinal benefits. Its roots, leaves, fruits, stems and seeds are used as an anti-inflammatory and helps with the reduction of rhinitis symptoms.[5]

Urtica dioica: It is commonly known as Nettle leaf. A clinical trial in 98 humans has shown that Nettle was highly effective against symptoms of allergies.[6]

Turmeric: It is an ancient herb used in giving color and flavor to food. Its main medicinal effects are anti-inflammatory, anti-allergic and anti-oxidant. Curcumin is an active component in Turmeric, which imparts an immuno-modulatory effect in reducing allergy symptoms. The anti-inflammatory effects also help in reducing redness and itchiness caused in severe allergic rhinitis. Many clinical trials have found the botanic to be highly effective. [7]

Circulation, Headaches And Migraines

> My son give me your heart, And let your eyes observe my ways.
> Proverbs 23:26

Rosemary: It is known as anthos. It is an analgesic which is a pain reliever, according to clinical trials. The soothing nature of rosemary oil supports the reduction of headaches, migraines and inflammation.[8]

Lavender: It not only soothes normal to mild headache, but also migraines due to its calming aroma according to clinical trials.[9]

Cayenne pepper: It is capsicum, red pepper or chilies. Clinical trials show that it significantly desensitizes pain sensation in cluster headaches.[10]

Nausea And Vomiting

> For when I am weak, then I am strong.
> 2 Corinthians 12:10

Andrographis paniculate (AP):
This King of Bitters has been used for centuries for reducing symptoms and speeding recovery. According to researchers, it did stop common cold and flu progression in several clinical cases. Today, it is getting more attention as a therapy against influenza due to a recent study that showed its effectiveness of inhibiting H1N1 Swine Flu [11]. Asia, America and Africa have used the plant to treat other conditions as well[12]. These conditions are vast: [13] Bronchitis, Cancer, Colic, Diabetes, Dysentery, Dyspepsia, Flatulence, High blood pressure, Leprosy, Skin diseases, Ulcers and Malaria.

Ginger: Human trials have shown that ginger is indeed an effective herb in reducing symptoms of nausea and vomiting. The rhizome or roots are anti-emetic, anti-spasmodic, and anti-microbial. This is especially useful with a soothing and cooling effect. Researchers have also found ginger helpful in reducing symptoms of cough and cold, and managing chronic disorders like high blood pressure, diabetes and soothing digestive problems[14].

Fennel: The seed is the part where the botanic is extracted. It has strong anti-microbial, anti-emetic and soothing properties which help in reducing symptoms of vomiting. Researchers have shown that fennel is an effective botanical for vomiting and nausea symptoms[15].

Lavender: Is a native to Europe regions, and known as Lavandula angustifolia. It has an incredible aromatic scent. The plant extract is used in making essential oil, concentrated with the active ingredients. But it's also found in many cosmetics and hygiene products. Lavender is beneficial for reducing the feeling of nausea and can help slow down or stop vomiting. Numerous studies have shown that it is effective[16].

Cinnamon: It is an effective botanic against vomiting, especially for morning sickness because of its anti-emetic and anti-spasmodic properties. Numerous clinical trials have found positive results for cinnamon[17].

Lemon: It is a very common citrus fruit widely used in cuisines around the world. The extract has large amounts of vitamin C and antioxidants. It has antiemetic effects. The aroma itself can reduce the feeling of nausea and vomiting[18].

Peppermint: It is native to the United States of America, Europe and the Middle East. It is known as Mentha piperita. The active compound is extracted from the leaves of the plant. Among all its beneficial properties, it is highly effective in relief of symptoms related to the digestive system problems. It relaxes the stomach muscles and has an antiemetic effect thus reducing vomiting. It is especially helpful in motion sickness. Numerous research on humans have proved the efficacy of the herb in reducing symptoms of vomiting[19] and treating vomiting, especially in pregnancy[20].

Cumin: The seeds are carminative, and soothing. It's used for treating gastrointestinal problems. Studies have proven that it is helpful in reducing nausea[21].

Clovers: It is native to Sri Lanka. It is known as Syzygium aromaticum. It's a beneficial herb well-known for their antiseptic and antimicrobial properties. It helps to reduce vomiting, including infections and reduce inflammation. Different studies on human have proven the effectiveness of this botanic[22].

Indigestion, Flatulence And Constipation

> However, the report went around concerning Him all the more; and great multitudes came together to hear, and to be healed by Him of their infirmities.
> Luke 5:15

Ginger: The botanic has been used effectively for soothing and calming intestinal spasms and other problems. It's the gingerol in ginger that promotes the anti-inflammatory and soothing effect on the intestinal wall. It also helps to reduce flatulence and excess gas accumulated in the stomach. This happens by stimulating digestion and increasing the passing of stool.[23]

Turmeric: It is well-known for its antibacterial, anti-inflammatory and antioxidant properties. It's also beneficial for helping to reduce gas accumulation in the stomach. There are numerous clinical trials among humans, which have shown the effectiveness of it on intestinal gas, motility and digestion.[24]

Dill: It is known by the Vikings as dilla. The botanical name is Shatapushpa. It is very popular as an anti-gas supporter. It is known for its carminative properties which help in removing trapped gas from the digestive track while working to lessen further complications.[25]

Cumin: It is native to Egypt. It's known as Jiraka. The dried fruit and seeds are used for spices and medicinal purposes. The active component is terpenoids. Studies have shown it helps with digestion and intestinal motility and reduction of flatulence.[26][27]. Studies have also shown the active component helps increase the rate of digestion. Especially increasing the secretion of bile, and better fat metabolism, reduction of flatulence, spasms and pain during digestion[28].

Fennel: The botanic is known as Marathon. The seed has been used to freshen the breath after eating and ease digestion. The tea form is also an excellent carminative that supports elimination of gas. Fennel is supported in many clinical trials which have shown it to be a highly effective herb for flatulence[29]

Mint: The botanic is known as Mentha. It is one of the most common flavoring agents found in our food industry. It is a common medicinal plant which helps in reducing intestinal problems and symptoms. It is especially effective in irritable bowel disease and flatulence. Research has shown its effectiveness against these problems[30].

Rosemary: It is a wonderful botanic for helping to fight inflammation of the colon. Researchers have shown it has anti-colitis properties which has helped in the reduction of intestinal gas as well[31].

Armor of God

Constipation: Throughout history, these foods and herbs have shown benefit in supporting the body against constipation.

1. Okra[32] Note (stewed or raw mixed in a smoothie is ideal) 2. Collard Greens[33]	3. Kiwi Fruit[34] [35] 4. Prunes[36] 5. Figs[37] 6. Senna[38] 7. Psyllium[39]

Fatigue And Exhaustion

But they that wait upon the Lord shall renew their strength; they shall mount up with wings as eagles; they shall run, and not be weary; and they shall walk, and not faint.
Isaiah 40:31

CoQ10: Coenzyme Q10 is the most important enzyme for good cellular health. It feeds the mitochondria, the "power plants" of the cells. Mitochondria produce 90% of the cellular energy required by the human body. Researchers have connected, moderate and severe fatigue with dysfunction of the mitochondria and decrease of energy production at a cellular level[40].

Ashwagandha: It is known as Withania somnifera or Indian ginseng. It is native to Africa and Asia and has been used throughout the world for centuries. The main chemical compounds are alkaloids, which help in increasing cognitive function and reducing mental confusion. Research on humans and animals helped establish the positive effects on neurodegenerative diseases. [41]

Cacao: It is native to Peru. It is known as Theobtoma. The dark unsweetened chocolate is not only a treat but has shown support for reducing many symptoms of illnesses. The active ingredients are extracted from the dried seeds of this plant which are flavonoids. Chocolates can regulate neurotransmitters, which help to stabilize mood and reduce fatigue. Trials on humans have concluded that cacao extracts can reduce symptoms of chronic fatigue syndrome[42].

Ginkgo biloba: It is native to China and known as maidenhair tree. The botanic is extracted from the leaves. The active components are flavonoids and terpenoids, addition to antioxidants. According to clinical trials, together they prevent damage to tissues in the central nervous system. It also offers a range of health benefits that help to improve mental health. Studies have shown its highly effective against mental confusion and helps promote clarity of the mind[43].

Muscle Pain And Soothing Support

> Now unto him that is able to do exceeding abundantly above all that we ask or think, according to the power that worketh in us.
> Ephesians 3:20

Ginger: It consists of compounds that inhibit the release of inflammatory substances which helps in reducing inflammation as well as soothing muscle pain. There are many scientific literatures which supports the effectiveness of ginger on muscle pain. One clinical trial found that ginger dietary supplements helped in the reduction of muscle pain caused by exercise.[44] [45]

Turmeric: It is the root of the plant belonging to the ginger family. Turmeric is an extremely potent herb which has anti-inflammatory, analgesic and antiseptic properties. In modern era, researchers have conducted thousands of clinical trials which have proven the effectiveness of turmeric in soothing muscle pain.[46]

Chamomile: It has analgesic, antispasmodic and anti-inflammatory properties and has been used to help reduce the cause and symptoms of muscle pain. Chamomile is especially effective in reduction of post-operative sore throat which was researched by Kyokong et al in the clinical trials[47].

Ginseng: It is native to eastern North America. It is known as Panax quinquefolius. It is widely cultivated in China. It is an ancient herb having potent properties that range from reducing symptoms of memory loss and muscle pain. Clinical trials have proven ginseng to be effective in helping muscle pain, damage and inflammation.[48] [49]

Capsicum: It's cayenne pepper and is found in red peppers or chilies. It is native to South America. It helps to reduce muscle pain by numbing the area and helps in reduction of inflammation. Numerous clinical trials have found capsaicin to be effective in reduction of neck pain, peripheral neuropathy and chronic pain.[50][51]

Epsom Salt Baths and Foot Soak: It is a mineral compound consisting of several electrolytes, including magnesium which has many health benefits. Epsom bath soak is highly popular for pain and muscle relaxation. The salts are a method used for pain reduction, which is effective in chronic pain. It has been used historically against neuropathic pain in cancer patients. Trials in both humans and animals has helped support the effectiveness of Epsom salt in pain reduction. [52][53]

White Willow Bark: It is native to Bulgaria. It is known as Bi Liu or Salix Alba. It is a potent herb which has been used for centuries for reduction of pain. It acts by inhibiting various compounds that cause inflammation in the body thus reducing pain. Researchers have conducted numerous trials which have proven the herb to be effective and safe against muscle pain[54] [55] [56].

Cinnamon: It has anti-inflammatory and antioxidant properties. Research in clinical trials has shown that cinnamon was effective in reducing of muscle pain and soreness when consumed daily[57].

Insomnia, Nervousness And Anxiety

For with God nothing shall be impossible.
Luke 1:37

Kava Kava: It is native to the South Pacific and is well known for its medicinal properties. The extracts from Kava contains kavalactones, which have GABAergic effects. Researchers have done clinical trials on humans and animals and concluded that Kava is effective in helping with sleep disturbances especially by calming the mind[58].

Lavender: It has special effects of calming the central nervous system. Several studies have determined the effectiveness in reducing insomnia and increasing duration of sleep[59].

St. John's Wort: It is commonly known as Hypericum perforatum. It is a plant native to Europe, America and Asia. It is used for the soothing and calming of the mind. Numerous trials have proven its effectiveness for relief of mild to moderate sleep disturbances. It acts on the nervous system, including the different pathways in the brain[60].

Valerian: It is known as Valeriana officinalis. It is a common herb which is native to Europe, North America and Asia. The active compound is extracted from the root and has anti-anxiety effects. It is mainly used as a botanic for helping with many health problems which includes mental disorders, anxiety, depression, sleep disturbances, and insomnia. There have been many trials which show the effectiveness of valerian root extract for helping with insomnia. The study found that "patients taking valerian had an 80% greater chance of reporting improved sleep compared with patients taking placebo[61]."

Dill: It helps with sleep regulation and calming and relaxing the mind and helping to induce proper sleep.[62]

Lemon balm: It is native to the United States of America, Europe and Asia. It is known as Melissa, or Bee balm. The botanic is beneficial for the heart, liver, diabetic health, mental health, wellbeing and defense against infections. Clinical trials on humans have shown it to be effective in reducing insomnia and sleep disorders as well[63].

Chamomile: It has been used as a botanic for thousands of years. It is a flowering plant native to the northern hemisphere. The botanic is mainly extracted from the flowers of the plant. The tea has relaxing properties and has been used for different disorders, including insomnia or sleep disturbances, depression and anxiety. Clinical trials have shown that chamomile is a highly effective sleep inducer[64].

Passionflower: It is native to the United States of America. It is known as Passiflora. It is a common herb used for anxiety and sleep disorders. Its active components have a soothing effect on the mind and the central nervous system. Clinical trials on humans has shown the extracts of this herb is effective in reduction of nervousness and anxiety, calming the mind, prolonging sleep and helping with mood changes[65].

Severe Anxiety, Stress, And Nerve Pain

> Inasmuch as there is none like You,
> O Lord (You are great, and Your
> name is great in might).
> Jeremiah 10:6

Chamomile: It is an ancient herb used all over the world for anxiety, nervousness and sleep disorders. It has been used for anti-inflammatory and anti-cancer support. Randomized controlled trials on human has shown that chamomile has an effect on the nervous system sleep latency and night time awakening without having any side effects. It's especially helpful in reducing severe anxiety [66] [67].

Kava Kava: The active component in the extract is kavapyrones. This compound has a relaxing and soothing effect on the human nervous system and the effects helps in reducing nervousness, and anxiety. Trials on humans have shown the effectiveness in reducing nervousness and severe anxiety[68].

Lavender: It is commonly used for its effectiveness in helping with relaxation, anxiety and nervousness. There have been trials on animals and humans where lavender extracts have helped these symptoms, including supporting mental wellbeing. Another clinical trial concluded that it helped reduce severe anxiety[69] [70] [71] [72].

Rosemary: The oil extract is soothing and has shown to reduce stress levels and anxiety in clinical trials.[73]

Valerian root: It calms the mind and regulates mood. There have been many clinical trials within the last three decades on both humans and animals that showed how valerian's botanic properties help to reduce nervousness[74].

Fennel: It is a widely used herb in cuisines throughout the world. It is mainly native to the Mediterranean countries, but available worldwide. Among medicinal properties, it is commonly known for its anti-anxiety effects, especially post pregnancy and postmenopausal. A trial among postmenopausal women showed a significant difference in anxiety among the study participants[75].

Ashwagandha: It is one of the most natural and easily available herbs worldwide. It is an adaptogen and helps to balance the different systems of the body. Especially hormones and helping to regulate sleep. Researchers have also identified that it helps with the reduction of stress and severe anxiety[76].

Lemon balm: The medicinal benefits include, cardio protection, hepato-protection (liver), anti-anxiety, anti-bacterial and anti-diabetic properties. Clinical trials on humans have shown the herb to be effective in reducing nervousness, stress and anxiety[77].

Skullcap: It is native to the United States of America. It is known as Blue skullcap or Scutellaria laterifolia. Clinical trial research has proven positive effects against anxiety. In many cases, this has been reported to be one of the best botanicals for people who experience severe anxiety along with restlessness, muscle tension, and jaw clenching[78][79].

Cinnamon: It is native to Asia. It is known as Cinnamomum burmanni. Studies have proven it helps regulate mood and balance anxiety[80].

Cayenne Pepper: Researchers have proven the effectiveness of cayenne helping to reduce neuralgia **(nerve pain)**, and fibromyalgia pain.[81]

Seizures / Epilepsy

Who is this King of glory? The Lord of hosts, he is the King of glory. Selah. Psalm 24:10

Kava Kava: It has been used throughout history for helping with anxiety, pain, and seizures. A clinical trial conducted on 101 individuals has found the herb to be effective in the treatment of the symptoms of seizures. Six compounds from the extract of the root demonstrated pharmacological effects and found that the herb's actions block the chemical compounds which may give rise to seizures[82].

Lavender: It is a wonderful botanic. Numerous trials have shown the oil vapor is highly effective in reducing the duration of seizures. Scientifically, the elements in the botanic blocks the glutamate induced neurotoxicity[83].

Rosemary: It has many medicinal effects that help fight seizures. Clinical trials on animals have revealed to be effective in increasing the latency period between two seizure attacks. The study has also revealed it helps to decrease the severity of seizures[84][85].

Gotu kola: It has had numerous animal studies that have proven its effectiveness as an antiepileptic botanic. It acts by affecting the GABAergic system.[86][87][88]

Skullcap: It is a common ancient antiepileptic herb. According to clinical trials, the flavonoid from the extracts have been used to act on the GABA receptors in the human nervous system for reducing seizures[89].

Mood And Depression

> And will be a Father unto you, and ye shall be my sons and daughters, saith the Lord Almighty.
> 2 Corinthians 6:18

Chamomile: It is native to Europe and Asia. It is known as Matricaria recutita. It is a flowering plant and has been used as a tea botanic for centuries. It's especially famous for its relaxing properties on the nerves. Clinical trials have shown that chamomile is a highly effective antidepressant and anti-anxiety agent[90].

Eschscholzia californica: It is native to California, and southwestern USA. It is known as California poppy. It is a flowering plant that consists of several active compounds that clinical trials have revealed it inhibiting and reducing symptoms of depression. Other reviews and trials conducted shown promising results for depression[91].

Ginkgo biloba: Its flavonoids and terpenoids are the active components extracted from the leaves of the plant. Its antioxidants give protection against oxidative damage to cells of the human body. Studies have shown it to be highly effective in lowering depression levels in humans [92] and helping to improve mental health[93].

Kava Kava: It is native to Vantuatu – the South Pacific (Oceania and east of Australia). It is known as yangona, awa, or piper methysticum. Clinical trials on humans and animals has shown Kava is effective in reducing anxiety and depression[94] [95].

Saffron: It is native to Spain. It is known as Spanish saffron or true saffron. It is a floral herb that not only has a beautiful aroma, but also has the nutritive properties of relaxing and balancing the mood. Its effect on mental wellbeing are promising. Five controlled trials on humans have proven that saffron was able to reduce symptoms of depression in adults[96] [97].

St. John's Wort: It is known as Hypericum perforatum. It has been the most common herb used for depression throughout history. Trials have proven its effectiveness for relief of mild to moderate mental health problems including depression. The active ingredients hypericin and hyperforin are the compounds that have the antidepressant effect.[98] [99]

Valerian root: It is native to Europe, North America and Asia. This herb is commonly used for mental health, particularly for its positive anti-anxiety effects. The active compound is extracted from the root. There have been many clinical trials showing the effectiveness of it reducing depression and anxiety[100].

Mental Confusion And Mental Fatigue

> And I heard, as it were, the voice of a great multitude, as the sound of many waters and as the sound of mighty thunderings, saying, "Alleluia! For the Lord God Omnipotent reigns!
> Revelation 19:6

Ginkgo biloba: Ginkgo biloba is one of the most versatile herb which grows mainly in China. The botanic is extracted from the leaves of the plant. The active components of the botanic are flavonoids and terpenoids. It also contains antioxidants which together with the active ingredients inhibit damage of the tissues in the central nervous system. Additionally, it offers a range of health benefits for improving mental health. Studies have shown the herb to be highly effective in helping individuals with dementia, mild cognitive impairment and mental confusion[101].

Lavender: It is especially effective in calming the mind, and it is anti-anxiety and antidepressant. Several animal and human studies have determined the effectiveness of lavender in helping with mental health problems for example, mental confusion, especially at an older age[102].

Rosemary: It has been used throughout history as an effective botanic against mental problems, stress, anxiety, stomach problems, and infections. Researches have revealed the extracts of Rosemary and lavender are effective in against short-term memory[103].

Ashwagandha: It is known as Winter cherry. It helps in increasing cognitive function and lessening mental confusion. Researchers have established the effects of it helping to improve memory and cognitive functions[104].

Ginseng: It is extracted from the roots of the plant. Its antioxidative activities support cells getting an ample amount of oxygenation from the bloodstream, whereas, hypoxia is the opposite of cells getting oxygenation. Oxygen helps support proper functioning of neurotransmitters, but also improves cognition function. It's also used to build stronger memory, ease headaches, tinnitus, fight cardiovascular diseases or coronary heart disease. Numerous researchers have tested ginseng and concluded its effectiveness against neurodegenerative disease, including mental confusion[105].

Gotu kola: It is native to Asia. It is known as Indian Pennyworth, Centella asiatica or Brahmi. It is a perennial herbaceous shrub and is known for its positive effects on the brain and human health. Research has been numerous on humans, conducting the effectiveness of the botanica for helping with mental confusion and enhancing memory[106]. The active compounds are known as bacosides. The main component is extracted from the rounded small leaves and the tender stems. It acts by having an inductive effect on the GABA-ergic system which can stimulate or block neurotransmitters. That is why it has been found to support several neurodegenerative disorders.

Fighting Infections

For all infections I use Colloidal Silver, the formula is called Silver Shield w/Aqua Sol (20 ppm). For more information, see my herb store, www.NaturalHealthEdu.com. This formula that I use does not build-up in the skin or turn the skin blue (argyria) because the patented way in which it is processed. This Silver Shield is bioavailable pure silver nanoparticles that are suspended in pure water. My skin has never turned blue after using this Silver Shield, and I have been using it for years. If I was allergic to Silver, I could not use it.

It is a fact throughout history, Silver has been used for emergency purposes, and to replace antibiotics when appropriate. Although Colloidal Silver has been used to increase the effectiveness of some antibiotics according to PubMed.gov. The FDA, however, does not approve colloidal silver as a dietary supplement, even though it is commonly used in medicine and medical devices.

The medical profession uses it for wound dressings, antibacterial bandages, Antibacterial creams, X-Ray Films, Catheters, Endotracheal tubes, Cardiac devices, and Antiseptics, including eye drops for conjunctivitis and other eye infections.

In my practice, we use Silver Shield to deactivate mold and fungus in the lungs, skin infections, strep throat, stomach viruses, ear, eye and respiratory, sinus infections and more.

In the Bible Moses Used this Method

The book of Exodus 32:18-20, tells us Moses used the health benefits of gold as we do colloidal silver today. He took the golden calf and crushed it down into a powder to keep the Israelites from worshiping the calf. He mixed the powder in water and made the Israelites drink it. The gold's purity purified their bodies from infection due to it being an antiviral, antibacterial, and anti-fungal. That meant it killed or weakened both viruses and bad bacteria.

Today, antibiotics kill both good and bad bacteria but not viruses. That is why we use Silver Shield as a supernatural antibiotic because it dismantles the DNA of both viruses and bad bacteria. Incredibly, it does not dismantle the DNA of good bacteria. Therefore, it complements the immune system.

Emotional Balance For Courage

Support for the emotional balance for courage is a group of botanical flowers found in a dietary supplement liquid. For clinical references and more wellness benefits, please visit my herb store NaturalHealthEdu.com.

The Be Courageous Liquid Formula Helps With

• Vented fear	• Confidence
• Courage	• Better focus

It supports emotional balance in encouraging self-responsibility, building courage, confidence and helping with overwhelming fear. The adrenals are the organs that can help balance fear, but when the adrenals are stressed and hungry, it can become a challenge for them to balance stress levels and fear.

Some of the flowers in Be Courageous are Mountain Pride, Aspen, Scleranthus, Mimulus and Cerato.

The Be-Response-Able Formula Helps With

• Being able to respond • Suppressed fear	• Accountability • Audacity • Inner strength

Some of the flowers in Be-Response-Able are Black Eyed Susan, Milkweed, California Poppy, and Agrimony.

Emotional Balance For Grief

These flower essences help the body vent grief or suppressed fear. The lungs are what controls the grieving process. If a person holds onto grief longer than they should, the respiratory tract can be affected and the healing process as well.

The Release It Liquid Formula Helps With

• Vented grief • Grieving process • Letting go the past	• Emotional pain • Agony • Co-dependent

Some of the flowers in Release it is Self-Heal - Prunella vulgaris, Love Lies Bleeding, Chicory, Bleeding Heart, Chrysanthemum, Borage, and Star Thistle.

The Open Heart Liquid Formula Helps With

• Suppressed grief • Locked emotions	• Love / affection • Healing & joy

Some of the flowers in Open Heart are California Wild Rose, Baby Blue Eyes, Yerba Santa, Star Tulip, Evening Primrose, Pink Monkey flower, and Golden Ear Drops.

Emotional Balance For Anger

These are flower essences that support individuals who chronically repress or vent anger. It encourages a feeling of emotional wellness.

The Find Strength Liquid Formula Helps With

• Suppressed anger • Helplessness	• Low-self esteem • Fear

Some of the flowers in Find Strength are Mariposa Lily, Pine, Scarlet Monkeyflower, and Centaury.

The Keep Cool Liquid Formula Helps With

• Vented anger • Irritation	• Hostility • Easily aggravated

Some of the flower in the formula are Calendula, Snapdragon, Impatiens, Grape Vine, and Willow. The liver helps to balance anger, but when the liver is under chronic nutritional stress, healing processes can be delayed.

Emotional Balance For Stress

They are flowers that help support mental, emotional and physical stress.

Distress Remedy Liquid

• Mental and emotional stress • Trauma • Shock	• Crises • Low-self esteem • Uneasiness • Hopelessness

The flower liquids are Arnica, Star of Bethlehem, Rock Rose, Impatiens, Clematis, Cherry Plum and Red Clover.

4 Elimination Systems of The Body

These organs are the Circulation, Immune, Skin and Colon. They depend on each other during the detox process. It is important to know how these systems work together so you will know what may be hindering you from feeling better. When the organ functions are underactive or overpopulated with waste, it will slow down the healing process and delay it.

Therefore, they function better when they are unblocked from the stress.

Circulation and Immune

Light trampoline jumping is beneficial for these systems. It provides excellent support for anti-aging, toxin elimination, weight control, pain and promotes wellbeing. Truly, good circulation is the key! BouncingForHealth.com discussed the health benefits of trampoline jumping, stating that it supports the circulatory and respiratory system which also helps circulation in other organs.

Light trampoline jumping forces lymph fluid to move throughout the body. Movement is the only way to get lymph fluid moving. Deep breathing also moves lymphatic fluid, especially in the respiratory tract.

Exercising Lymph

A sweaty activity gets lymphatic fluid eliminating waste faster, which in-turn helps the bloodstream eliminate the waste. Exercising, walking, bike riding, tennis and other sports help the lymphatic system. Water is in heavy demand by every organ, tissue and cell in the body. It too also helps the movement of lymphatic fluids. Lymph needs to be moving to speed up the healing process.

Infrared Sauna

The infrared sauna forces blood-flow to the surface and then skin pores open and excrete environmental toxins and other unwanted substances. Perspiration is the key, and infrared saunas stimulates it very well. The infrared sauna makes rays that are similar to sun rays, but without UV radiation or extreme heat like the sun. The skin does not burn. However, a dry skin brush is good to unblock skin pores first.

On March 24, 2009 on Oprah.com, Dr. Oz talked about how infrared sauna therapy can enhance blood flow, lower high blood pressure, burn calories, ramp-up metabolism and eliminate toxins effectively.

Epsom

Epsom salt baths are a great way to mildly detox the body. Epsom salt has the mineral magnesium sulfate, which attracts water and pulls water and tiny substances out of the skin pores. Most substance that's water-soluble and is tiny enough can pass through the skin while detoxing with Epsom salt. For more benefits of Epsom salt, see The Epsom Salt Council at Epsomsaltcouncil.org

On Doctor Oz's website, they discussed how Epsom salt is a good remedy to exfoliate, and treat small wounds, dry skin, sore muscles, swelling, inflammation, and fight illnesses.

Skin

When the skin pores are blocked with old encrusted debris, the pores are not at liberty to remove lymphatic waste efficiently. Then the circulating waste or toxins tend to accumulate into weaker organs, making them more vulnerable to challenges. That's why unblocking the pores can help speed up waste elimination from the body and boost the healing process.

Lymphatic Massage

It is a delicate massage that uses soft touch to glide lymphatic fluid under the skin and helps break up lymphatic congestion around the body. Massagetherapy.com discussed the benefits of lymphatic massages. They said it can help break-up sluggish tissues that are affected by stagnated waste and swelling problems. They said lymphatic massage is therapeutic to the body in several other ways too.

Dry Skin Brushing

One of the greatest advantages of Iridology is that the irises reveal locations where skin pores are blocked around the body. This also helps identify where to focus on for decongesting particular areas in the body.

On August 21, 2012, Huffington Post wrote an article on the benefits of dry skin brushing. They talked about it banishes cellulite and improves skin tone. They discussed the skin being the biggest organ of the body and how dry skin brushing helps to remove dead skin, boost circulation and lymphatic fluid drainage, as well as speeding up toxin removal from the body.

Colon

The blood in the colon travels to every organ and tissue in the body. Therefore, if the blood still has old circulating waste, then every organ and tissues will get that same blood-waste. This tends to promote organ weaknesses and set the beginning stages of diseases. Additionally, waste can impact and ferment or spoil inside areas of the colon wall. This can ultimately build into a weakness, and bacteria, viruses, and parasites can use those areas as a drainage point to excrete their waste. Infection and inflammation can also become a result, including colon diseases and other symptoms.

The good news is that all 4 Elimination Systems can be detoxed and unblocked with the right foods and dietary supplements – including the urinary and respiratory tracts which are 2 more essential elimination systems.

The Truth About Parasites And Recovery

• Sexually Transmitted Diseases -STDs • Spread by kissing • Uncooked meat • Insect bites • Infected pets • Infected soil • Infected raw vegetables	• Sharing infected needles • Infected drinking water • Hot springs • Hot tubs • Lakes • Ocean • Rivers • Swimming pools

| • Infected blood transfusions | |

Parasites create weakness in the body, and weakness creates an environment where sickness and disease can take root.

Parasites can thrive off life in the blood. *The life of all flesh is in the blood. - Leviticus 17:14.* Therefore, they can live in a person's bloodstream and small and large intestines. Including the brain, gall bladder, gall duct, kidneys, ureters, bladder, eyelashes, eyes, eyebrows, scalp, face, liver, heart, nose, nerves, muscles, lungs, spleen, pancreas, lymph nodes, hair follicles, and connective tissues[107] [108] [109] [110] [111] [112].

Some of the ways they do their damages is by eating the nutrients in a person's bloodstream and excreting waste into the bloodstream as well. If the infection is prolonged and not eliminating with the parasites and their eggs, they tend to promote severe illnesses.

Parasites are sexually transmitted and carry viruses. They are transmitted orally by kissing an infected person who has parasites in their saliva or blood. They can also enter the body through openings in the skin such as a wound, or from the nose or mouth.

Parasites that thrive off blood can be found in raw meat. Therefore, cooking all meats completely can reduce infection. The quality of a person's stomach acid determines if it kills the parasites and their eggs before they can travel to other organs. If stomach acid is sufficient enough, it will kill those pathogens, but if not, then they can slip through and infect the person's health.

Insects, such as ticks, mosquitos, sand flies and others blood sucking insects can carry parasites in their bloodstream and infect people who they bite.

Animals, including pets, wild animals can get infected with parasites too, especially because they do eat other animals, insects, or play or walk through areas where there's parasitic activity. Therefore, being around pets, hand washing with water and soap is key. Also deworming pets is essential.

Contaminated soil with infected animal feces is one of the many ways that both humans and pets get infected with parasites. For that reason, all humans should wear shoes walking on grass. In addition to sitting on benches or chairs while on the grass.

All raw fruits or vegetables should be washed thoroughly before eating. They have potential contamination with infected animal feces because vegetation grows in soil.

Infected persons that donate blood or share their syringe needles can transfer parasites this way and other diseases. Drinking water that's contaminated is another way that parasite transferred into an individual or pet.

People can get infected with parasites from sitting in hot springs, hot tubs, or swimming pools, walking in inside ponds, lakes, oceans, or rivers.

Parasites can be indicative of the following symptoms if chronic – however, the correct diagnostic test (cultures from saliva, stool, urine, skin, or intestinal barium or other pathogen diagnostic test) can help give a positive diagnosis.

• Abdominal bloating
• Abdominal cramping
• Aches and pains
• Anemia
• Chronic allergies
• Chronic bad breath / odor
• Blood in stool
• Blood in cough
• Chronic burping
• Chronic fatigue
• Chronic flatulence
• Chronic muscle ache
• Crohn's disease
• Fever
• Foul smelling stool	• Itchy anus
• Itchy nose
• Itchy skin
• Heart burn
• IBS
• Leaky gut / intestinal permeability
• Loss of appetite
• Malnutrition
• Nausea / vomiting
• Unexplained pale skin
• Skin infections
• Skin lesions / rash
• Sleeping challenges
• Unexplained weight loss / weight gain
• Viral infections

These foods and herbs have been used throughout history and have shown beneficial against parasites, their eggs, and similar pathogens[113][114][115][116][117][118][119][120][121][122][123].

1. Probiotics 2. Basil 3. Colloidal silver (it must be processed correctly first) 4. Black walnut	5. Wormwood 6. Pau D'Arco 7. Coconut oil 8. Euphorbia 9. Black cumin 10. Oregano oil

20 Things That Weaken The Gut

1. Artificial food chemicals 2. Artificial perfumes 3. Antibiotics, steroids 4. Heavy metals in the body 5. Parasites 6. Fungus, viruses 7. yeast overgrowth 8. Microwaving food 9. Excess wheat diet	10. Toxins in the bloodstream 11. Poisons in the bloodstream 12. Chronic anxiety and stress 13. Excess simple Sugars 14. Excess dietary Fats 15. Allergies 16. Birth control pills 17. Tobacco/alcohol 18. Excess caffeine 19. EMF / Wi-Fi 20. Free-radicals

70-80% of our immunity is found in the digestive tract. All diseases begin in the gut. Along with all our organs, the gut is our brother's keeper, ready to defend us at all cost to stop disease and sickness from taking root in God's property. I'll repeat it. Our bodies are God's property and our organs treat it as such as it fights to protect us. God designed our organs to survive and live.

Disease thrives in a weakened body. That's why a healthy gut equals a healthy, successful recovery. It's astonishing how well the body does when strengthen with life and vitality – God's way! Disease and sickness can't keep up with that and for that reason has a hard time taking root to kill, steal and destroy. *The thief cometh not, but for to steal, and to kill, and to destroy: I am come that they might have life, and that they might have it more abundantly. John 10:10*

50 Things That Support The Gut

Our organs are held together by a protein molecule complex structure of 16,000 atoms. It's collagen, and not only does our skeletal structure depend on it but so does our gut wall. Collagen is fibrous connective tissues that are intestinal tissues, elastic tissues, fatty tissues, brain tissues, spinal cord tissues, skin, hair, nails, joints, tendons, ligament, and cartilage. Connective tissues surround each of our muscles too.

Animal broth is collagen (glutamine), which is one of the nutrients that can help build and repair[124] collagen in the body. We can get bone broth from animal bones by boiling it to extract the collagen, amino acids - proteins, and minerals like silica, magnesium, calcium, phosphorus, and sulfur. Amino acids are the building blocks of proteins. Without them our bodies could not produce cells and tissues for our organs to function. That is why glutamine, glucosamine and chondroitin are needed.

It's the connective tissues that protects[125] and hold together the gut wall, muscles, skin, teeth, hair, nails, joints, ligaments, tendons, and fibrous tissues.

Foods that Support Collagen Production

1. Aloe vera gel and liquid	10. Nuts and seeds 11. Olive oil 12. Pomegranate

2. Beta-glucan Foods 3. Bone broths 4. Cabbage 5. Cauliflower 6. Coconut 7. Copper foods 8. Green tea 9. Legumes	13. Proteins 14. Royal jelly 15. Silicon (silica) Foods 16. Sulfur food 17. Vitamin B foods 18. Vitamin K – leafy Greens 19. Zinc foods

Probiotics

Probiotics support the health of the gut friendly microflora[126]. The good news is the gut also naturally manufactures these. Probiotics kill bad bacteria, but so do antibiotics. However, antibiotics kill good bacteria and does not replace it[127]. That's why it has been reported that some people develop other symptoms after a round of antibiotics because they did not replenish their gut microflora with probiotics or enough probiotics.

Probiotics are an incredible resource. They populate and guard the small intestines, colon and the appendix. They build up the guts good bacteria and help create a defense against parasites, viruses and the overgrowth of damaging bacterial or yeast. Candida yeast is one of the main reasons why women get urinary tract infections. There are over 400 probiotic species. The most common are acidophilus and lactobacillus that fight for us. Not only are probiotics beneficial for the digestive tract, but also the immune system because it helps the immune system strengthen the gut. If an overgrowth of bad bacteria or pathogens does happen in the gut, a probiotic increase can help fight it and reduce its toxic effects from weakening the body.

The gut also manufactures vitamins when the body calls for it. For example, the beneficial bacteria can manufacture folic acid, biotin, riboflavin (B2), pantothenic acid (B5), pyridoxine (B6), and vitamin K. The body needs complex B vitamins because they feed organ systems; especially the brain and the nervous system. These vitamins have a calming effect to the brain and the nervous system. They are also known to boost energy, especially for slow metabolizers.

It is the Colony Forming Units (CFU) of probiotics that make up the count strains of probiotics in the food. Most probiotic foods have billions more colony forming units, then most dietary supplements on the market today. However, dietary supplements provide a quick source for critical care, and maintenance in daily use for good health - a true benefit to the body!

Prebiotics

Prebiotics tremendously help probiotics and the health of the gut[128][129][130][131]. Prebiotics are called FOS, or Fructo-Oligosaccaharides. These are carbohydrate fibers that don't digest in the gut, but instead ferment there so that beneficial bacteria can eat it and grow to populate the gut.

Here's more good news! Prebiotics aids calcium and inulin absorption, according to one clinical study done on animals. The Journal of Nutrition, and the American Journal of Clinical Nutrition found that both calcium and inulin (which is used to test kidney function) increased in absorption in the gut and bloodstream[132]. Inulin is fructan fiber which is a natural polysaccharide. It is found in vegetables, fruits and herbs.

Probiotics and Prebiotics traces are found in specific foods. Eating them raw gives the best health effects. Probiotic Food sources are found in fermented foods and this list shows some of them. The Beets can be fermented and that will allow the beneficial bacteria to eat up the high sugar content. Beet sauerkraut or pickled beets can be found in specialty grocery stores.

Probiotic Foods

20. Beets	27. Sauerkraut miso soup; made with fermented rye, beans, rice or barley, (soy - but not ideal for estrogen dominance health issues or allergies)
21. Blue green algae	
22. Buttermilk (but not ideal for congestion issues)	
23. Coconut kefir	
24. Coconut milk	
25. Coconut yogurt	28. Kimchi
26. Cow Yogurt (but not ideal for congestion issues)	29. Pickles
	30. Red cabbage

Prebiotic Foods

31. Jerusalem artichokes	39. Tomatoes
32. Asparagus	40. Chicory root
33. Leeks	41. Unripe bananas

34. Garlic 35. Onions 36. Honey 37. Fruits and berries 38. Apple cider vinegar	42. Most greens (i.e. collard, kale, spinach) 43. Jicama 44. Yacon 45. Almonds

Larch is another fiber food that stimulates the proliferation of good bacteria like bifidobacteria and lactobacillus probiotics. They do this by stimulating the cell-to-cell growth of probiotics[133].

Prebiotic Larch Arabinogalactan Foods

46. Reishi mushroom - May not be ideal for yeast overgrowth or urinary tract infections. Although it has medicinal properties that support immunity, there is controversy whether it will feed yeast (Candida) or not.
47. Echinacea
48. Radish
49. Apple, plums
50. Carrots, cherries and tomatoes

Synthetic Sodium Nitrates (Salt)

Sodium Nitrate is salt used as a preservative for curing processed meats like packaged ham, turkey, smoked meats, jerky, hot dogs, sausages, corn beef, luncheons, and bacon.

There are natural nitrates that are found in herbs, spices and foods like spinach and lettuce. There is also pharmaceutics nitrates that dilate blood vessels. We consume more nitrates used for curing or preserving meats than ever, and when eating in excess, this tends to be harmful to the body. The nitrates for curing meats are synthetic chemicals.

Nitrates form a chemical bond with amino acids in the digestive tract and then converts into nitrosamine, a carcinogen, according to a clinical study by the Department of Preventive Medicine, State University of New York Health Science Center. The study was found in Cancer Epidemiol Biomarkers Prev. 4(1):29-36, 1995. It revealed evidence of nitrosamines being a dangerous, potent carcinogen with a high risk towards mouth, esophagus, larynx and breast cancers.

It's better to select meat products that says on the package, "uncured" and no nitrates. It is also good to know that animal fatty tissues are where pesticides, herbicides, chemicals, other toxins and foreign substances are mostly stored. Limiting this is healthwise. The more animal fat products consumed, the more chemical toxins ingested. Eating raw clams, oysters, or fish (sushi) is another way that can lead to health challenges if there the food is infected. Raw eggs too, unless you know a farmer who has healthy chickens.

Salt Choices

Salt comes from evaporated water from the ocean. It can also come from minerals from rocks.

Table Salt

It is refined salt with over 98% sodium chloride and 2% moisture absorbents and iodine. When table salt is processed, most of its minerals, vitamins and other nutrients are removed. But those minerals normally don't get thrown away. They are added to dietary supplements, food products or used for industrial purposes.

Research shows excess salt may cause other mineral depletions or excess in the human body. An article in Bone and Mineral Research said, "every 1,000 mg of table salt in the diet excrete 500 mg of calcium from the body." My guess is that excess salt excretes that calcium from the bones since the bones are the largest calcium reserves in the human body. When excess calcium leaves the bones, it can trigger bone loss and fractures.

Iodized Salt

It is a form of table salt mixed with low levels of potassium iodide (iodine).

Salt Substitute

This is made of (synthetic) potassium and chloride instead of sodium chloride, found in table salt.

Sea Salt (Unrefined Salt)

It is evaporated sea salt with no or little iodine, but has minute amounts of trace mineral. The removal of iodine happens during the drying process. The color of salt is a TELL-TELL sign of its rich nutrients of vitamins and minerals. Salt is supposed to be colorful. Iodine is available for people to help satisfy their thyroid and other organ system functions. It can be found naturally in sea vegetables, fish, black walnut botanical, pineapple, onions, lettuce, tomatoes, spinach, or specific iodine dietary supplement.

Himalayan (Unrefined)

It is crystal rock salt, found in the mines of the Punjab Region of Pakistan. This salt gets its pink color from iron oxide. It has a higher content of 82 trace minerals, including traces of iodine. Removal of impurities occur through natural processing.

Grey Salt (Unrefined)

It is Celtic sea salt, harvested from the pure clay linings of salt beds from the sea. Grey salt is better unrefined then refined because it has little preservatives or additives. It has a high mineral count with traces of iodine. Removal of impurities occur through natural processing also.

Bamboo Salt (Parched)

This salt is roasted sea salt and the impurities are removed through processing. The salt is poured into a bamboo cylinder that is packed with yellow mud. The mud is packed with minerals to give the salt more nutrients and flavor.

Hormone Disruptors

Xenoestrogens are endocrine (glandular) disruptors and they are found in pesticides, herbicides, plastics and some pharmaceuticals. Xenoestrogens affect our endocrine system. That system comprises of the prostate, and testes in males and ovaries in females. Also, the hypothalamus, thyroid, pineal, pituitary, parathyroid, adrenals and the pancreas and thymus. The pancreas, however is a gland and a digestive organ, while the thymus is both a gland and an immune system organ.

Xenoestrogens disrupts the biosynthesis or chemical balance of both human and animal hormones. Our hormones are natural chemical messages that are produced and secreted by the endocrine system. They select and direct the actions of every cell and organ system in our bodies. For example, they control our heart rate, sleep, mood, metabolism, body temperature, tissue function and growth and development of our organs from birth until we get old.

Xenoestrogens are fake estrogens that are linked to carcinogens, including breast cancer[134]. We come in contact with these every day. Xenoestrogens are industrial chemicals that are used in many consumer products. Not only are Xenoestrogens linked to cancers, but also other ailments, including infertility and babies born premature, with altered DNA, which leads to genetic birth defects.

Xenoestrogens PCBs

PCBs (polychlorinated biphenyls) are chlorine compounds found in wood floor finishes, paint, ink, adhesives, caulking, GMO, and some insecticides. PCBs have been banned in the United States in 1970, but are still in use in flame-retardants used to insulate electrical poles, transformers and capacitors, vacuum pumps, and hydraulic devices. Therefore, PCBs are still leaching into rivers, soil and our crops because of years of neglect and mis-handling of those electrical devices. At one time Monsanto used PCBs under the name Aroclor xxxx.

Today, Monsanto uses Roundup Ready a glyphosate herbicide to spray crops to kill weeds and insects. They also engineer synthetic seeds to grow GMO crops – which is a mix of unnatural and natural produce. It is toxic to health.

Xenoestrogens PBBs

PBBs (polybrominated biphenyls) are also flame-retardant PCBs. They are found in plastics used in electronic products like T.V. Sets, laptops, cell phones, and radios.

Xenoestrogens BPA

BPA (bisphenol A) is polycarbonate and epoxy chemicals. They are found in durable plastics products like plastic water bottles, DVDs, CDs, children's toys, baby pacifiers and teethers, some medical devices and dental sealants, plastic food containers, and lining the inside of canned foods and beverages, including canned baby formulas.

Xenoestrogens Phthalates

They are plasticizers and are used to make plastic and vinyl more flexible. They are used in a variety of consumer products including beauty care products like hair sprays, body lotions, soap, hair shampoo, conditioners, cosmetics, nail polish, perfumes. They are also used in plastic wrap, plastic food containers, household cleaning products, solvents, curtains, blinds, medical supplies and equipment.

Common pesticide is methoxychlor, chlorpyrifos, dichlorodi-phenyl-trichloro-ethane – DDT.

Xenoestrogen Fungicides (vinclozolin)

It is sprayed on vegetation to control mold, and rotting.

Xenoestrogen (die-thyl-stilbestrol – DES)

It is a pharmaceutical agents that is used as a birth control drug and hormonal replacement therapy drug.

Phytoestrogenic Foods Are Known To Help

Xenoestrogens will disrupt the hormonal system of the body after they have accumulated and populated the bodies estrogen receptor sites. The job of Phytoestrogenic foods is to get to the estrogen receptor sites first and populate the doorways to the cells so that xenoestrogens do not get enough space to attach to the doors of the cells. However, the body still has to work to get them out.

This list of foods is not comprehensive, but it gives you a general idea.

Phytoestrogenic Foods

1. Alfalfa	17. Licorice root
2. Anise	18. Mint
3. Apples	19. Mung beans
4. Barley	20. Oats
5. Beans	21. Pomegranates
6. Carrots	22. Red clover
7. Chickpeas	23. Rice
8. Coffee	24. Rice bran
9. Fennel and	25. Sage

10. Fenugreek	26. Sesame seeds
11. Flax seeds	27. Soybeans and soy products
12. Ginseng	
13. Hops	28. Tempeh
14. Kudzu	29. Wheat berries
15. Legumes	30. Wheat germ
16. Lentils	31. Yams

Phytoestrogens tend to help balance the body against many ailments and diseases, but with everything, it should be done with proper balance.

Soy

Most Soy is GMO now. That would make it xenoestrogens. But soy is also a phytoestrogen food.

Estrogenic Dominance

Research suggest people that are estrogenic dominant could have better hormonal balance by reducing Phytoestrogenic and estrogenic foods in their diet, because Phytoestrogens are still estrogens, but weaker ones. However, for women that are in menopause, these foods can be of great help to them. But with everything, moderation is key. Researchers have found that if progesterone the hormone that balances estrogen in the body is not in balanced, then estrogen dominance tends to occur.

Keep in mind that, by far, soy has the highest estrogen compound among all Phytoestrogenic foods.

Trick Food vs Organic Food

Nutrient Depleted Foods

1. Unbleached-enriched or enriched white flour
2. Empty calories
3. Low nutrients
4. Synthetic nutrients
5. The whiter the product, the bleached

When you are shopping for breads, flip to the label and read the ingredients. If it says *unbleached - enriched or just enriched,* then chances are it has low nutritious nutrients. These breads have empty calories; meaning, that they do have calories but are nutrient-poor. After organic foods have been eaten for a season or two, the body can tell the difference between organic, natural, and nutrient-poor foods. It's the taste buds that are the first to figure it out.

In these breads, the raw nutrients are removed during processing. But it is the raw nutrients that sustain the body. Manufacturers do add synthetic nutrients. They look to produce a certain quality and taste in the bread, For example, making it softer, lighter, whiter, or darker in color. They also enhance the flavor or reduce it for a desired taste. When the raw nutrients are taken, fewer health benefits are available to the body. This can lead to health challenges if eaten in excess. When the body is low in nutrients to support itself, a tendency towards organ stress and low energy arises. Organs need more energy just to battle artificial and toxic chemicals in order to trap, neutralize and safely escort them out of the body.

Unbleached Enriched Flour
This is whole grain flour and the raw nutrients are removed. Synthetic nutrients are added to make a finished product tastier, softer, or whiter.

Enriched Flour
This is bleached whole grain flour that also had its raw nutrients removed, and synthetic

nutrients added for a desired taste. Keep in mind that if the ingredients do not list a bleaching agent, like chlorine, or benzoyl peroxide, then the flour most likely been bleached. However, then it might say un-bleached-enriched, instead.

We all eat these foods from time to time. But what I do is include a multi-vitamin to supplement with that meal, or a fresh lemon mixed with water. I also eat vegetables with it to receive some raw nutrients. These help me bring balance back. But understand, multi-vitamins, even with good food is beneficial because food is only as good as the soil in which it was grown in. For example, if the soil is nutrient depleted, then the food will also be nutrient depleted.

Non-Nutrient Depleted 100% Wheat

1. All nutrients intact
2. Non-bleached
3. Natural taste
4. Best alternative

100% Whole wheat flour does not have its raw nutrients removed. It's not bleached with chemicals either. The texture is heavier, and the flavor is richer in taste. Unquestionably, 100% whole wheat is by far a better alternative to all nutrient depleted, bleached flour breads.

Reading Food Labels

Most of us have to read the nutritional facts on food labels. But how does one know how much of the food product is actually in the product? Descriptions can be misleading by up to 80%. That's why it is useful to read all the ingredients on the label. An example of an electrolyte sports drink that says "Orange," on the front, but the truth is, there's no orange juice in it. Instead the ingredients might say, "natural flavors or all-natural flavors." But it is a fact that the "natural flavors" could be MSG, a flavor enhancer. See the list of Toxic Food Ingredients in Resources and References.

The other way to read labels is to see where the main ingredients appear in the sentence. If the ingredient is closer to the first sentence in the paragraph, then that's a good sign that that food has what it says it has, otherwise, if the ingredient is listed last, then most likely it has less of that ingredient.

Processed Nutrient Depleted Foods

1. Refined foods
2. Refined oils
3. Instant foods
4. Low-fat and fat-free
5. Some Dehydrated foods
6. Flavored sauces / mixes
7. Ultra-pasteurized dairy products

Processed foods are white pasta, refined grains, and refined oatmeal products. Refined oils are processed at high temperatures, which makes them oxidized, rancid and a free radical themselves. Free radicals are known to inflame blood vessels, which has the potential to put a person at risk of inflammatory challenges. Refined oils are in canola oil, vegetable oils, Crisco®, soybean oil, corn oil, sunflower oil, safflower oil, and peanut oil. If the ingredients say "hydrogenated" then it is rancid!

Healthy oils that are not rancid will say cold pressed, unrefined, unfiltered, and have no hydrogenated or partially hydrogenated oils in America. Most baked pastries are baked with hydrogenated or partially hydrogenated oils – thus refined and rancid!

Packaged instant foods includes pre-flavored foods and instant white rice, low-fat and fat-free dieting products, unless it has multi-vitamin nutrition added. Some dehydrated products have no nutritious taste. This is a red flag that a majority of its nutrients might be removed. However, dehydrated foods processed by a good dehydrator processor will still leave the raw nutrients in the food intact. Keep in mind that some nutritious fluid is removed during processing, but the fiber is still there and can help the body recover. Dehydrated foods can be vegetables, fruits, nuts, seeds and spices.

Most canned foods, bottled sauces or flavored mixes are nutrient depleted if good nutrients were not added back. Cow dairy milk products that are ultra-pasteurized, pasteurized or homogenized are heated at high temperatures to destroy viruses and bacteria, but this also reduces minerals, active enzymes and proteins as well. Enzymes are needed in milk to help the consumers' stomach acid break down the milk's protein and sugar. Lactose intolerance has been helped with the enzyme, lactase, which is the enzyme that breaks down milk to where it's digestible.

When pasteurization occurs, it oxidizes the milk and free radicals form. Free radicals do damage to healthy living cells in the body.

Minimally Processed Products
1. Less altered food
2. No artificial flavor
3. No coloring ingredient
4. No chemical preservatives
5. No synthetic ingredient
6. No solvent extraction
7. No acid hydrolysis
8. No chemical bleaching

Minimally processed foods are less likely to have steroids, antibiotics or hormones. But there is no guarantee with changing regulations. The food package will usually state if it has these chemicals or not. The ingredients may say no artificial flavors, but then say natural flavors, however, natural flavors can still be MSG.

100% Natural Products

1. Not Organic	8. Steroid-Free
2. All Natural	9. Antibiotic-Free
3. No Artificial Colors	

4. No Artificial Chemicals 5. Free-Range 6. Cage-Free 7. Hormone-Free	10. Minimally Processed 11. Possibly Non-GMO 12. Possibly Organic Ingredients

Natural food does not mean organic, nor does it have the USDA organic seal. However, they can have organic ingredients- it will say that on the label. These foods are one step down from organic. Natural foods can be anything from animal products, nuts, grains, fruits, and vegetables. However, they can still be high in salt and sugar, even though the ingredients are as natural as possible. The labels may also say all natural, free-range, hormone-free, steroid-free, minimally processed, no artificial colors, or chemicals, and Non-Genetically Modified (Non-GMO).

GMO - Genetically Modified Organisms

1. Plant foods - genetically engineered
2. DNA changed
3. Engineered to enhanced color or taste
4. Engineered to resist viruses
5. Engineered to repel bugs
6. Pesticides used (Roundup Ready)

7. Added nutrients or removed nutrients

GMO or GM is plant foods derived from genetically modified organisms (GMO). This means that their DNA has been genetically changed by the insertion of genes or the deletion of genes. Some plants are genetically modified to resist pesticides with Roundup Ready, so the pesticides only kill the weeds and not the plant itself. Other plants are genetically modified to resist viruses. These are inserted with a protein gene of the virus. There are plants that are inserted with omega 3 genes, and other nutrient to make a specific food type.

No GMO foods are allowed in the organic farming systems, and if found, the food cannot be sold as organic. However, because of the USDA leniency in allowing GMO crops, organic regulations have been revised to allow foods with up to 0.9% GMO as of today. These foods can sell as organic and not have a GMO food label or GMO listed on the label. Nonetheless, organic farmers are doing the best job they can with all the regulations and costs they have to contend with.

Organic

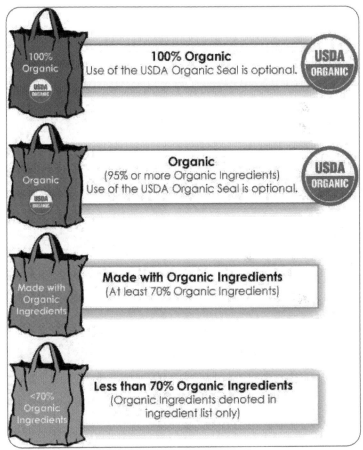

Source: U.S. Department of Agriculture

Organic Foods are BEST! – Especially for the sick, babies, children, pregnant women and the elderly. There are organic foods for nearly every food category, so look for foods that say organic or 100% Organic with the "USDA Organic" seal. Those foods are minimally processed and better for our organ systems.
Organic foods are supposed to be free of radiation, antibiotics, pesticides, herbicides, hormones, steroids, Genetically Modified Organism (GMO) artificial preservatives and food colorings and dyes.

The United States Department of Agriculture (USDA) certifies third-parties to monitor the food production of organic foods. They make sure it was not grown with conventional pesticides, artificial fertilizers, human waste, sewage sludge, radiation or irrigation which is artificial water. In order for food products to receive a USDA Organic seal the manufacturers must abide by these standards.

Free Range vs. Cage Free Produce

1. Ethical environments
2. Outdoors
3. Stocking densities
4. Greater feed selections

5. Healthier chickens
6. May not be hormone, antibiotic or steroid free

Animal products that say Free Range means that the animal had access to the outdoors - weather permitting, and the farm was held below certain stocking densities. This means that they were raised in a more ethical environment. Chickens eat flax seeds; which has Omega-3 and proteins. They eat other seeds, nuts, fruits, vegetables, grass and bugs of course. The good thing is that they tend to lay eggs with a higher Omega-3 content than those animals feed corn and soy. On the labels, look for antibiotic, hormone and steroid free.

Produce: Antibiotic, Hormones, Steroids

Here's the problem. When animals are sick, the veterinarian orders treatment, and the animal is administered antibiotics. The downside is when we eat the same animal products or something with its ingredients, if the antibiotics remained in the animal's body, we ingest a minute amount of it too. The bad news is when we eat these in excess, their antibiotics eventually affects our health too.

Organic farmers adapt to holistic methods wherever and wherever possible. However, if antibiotics are necessary, on the advice of the veterinarian, they must give that animal antibiotics. The animal product will not be sold as organic in that case. But the label could say steroid or hormone-free if that's the case.

Estrogen
Excess estrogen hormones are another concern. They are growth hormones that are anabolic in nature, meaning that they build up tissues, creating more tissue growth. It becomes a problem when out of control. Excess has been linked to abnormalities like cyst, lumps, bumps, and tumors - including benign fibroids. One of the reasons why farmers inject their animals with estrogen is to make a better profit on sales. Farmers make more money if the animals are fatter and heavier.

For some humans' reproductive organs have a higher risk of being affected by excess estrogen. Estrogen receptor sites are in reproductive organs too. Studies show that persons with estrogen dominant bodies have a higher risk of developing benign uterine fibroids, fibrocystic breasts, breast cancer and other risk factors. However, the counter hormone progesterone is used to balance estrogen and reduce estrogen dominance. The body makes progesterone, but too much can also lead to health challenges. The good news is excess estrogen can be detoxed out. The American Cancer Society stated that "for women who still have a uterus, doctors generally prescribe estrogen and progesterone therapy. Progesterone is needed because estrogen alone can increase the risk of cancer of the uterus."

Steroids
Synthetic Steroids are another type of synthetic hormone that animals are injected with to suppress or decreases swelling in their bodies. It's healthwise to choose meats that say steroid, hormone, and antibiotic free, or 100% Organic with a USDA Organic stamp.

Grass-Fed Animals: Produce

1. Organic	5. Minerals, vitamins
2. No food dyes	6. Omega 3
3. Quality protein	7. Healthiest
4. Antioxidants	

Grass Fed

Grass fed animal meats can come from goats, lambs, bison, cows, sheep, dairy and chickens (including their eggs). These animals are typically organic, steroid, antibiotic and hormone free. They have no added synthetic colors, and are quality proteins, higher antioxidants, minerals, vitamins, and omega 3.

Wild Caught Fish vs Farm Raised

Wild Caught Fish

1. Freely swim	6. No pesticides
2. Lesser diseased	7. No steroids
3. Higher omega 3	8. No dyes
4. Quality protein	9. Low xenoestrogen
5. No antibiotics	

Wild caught fish are not caged. They can freely swim about. They are wild caught, processed and sold on the market. They are less diseased prone, but mercury can still be an issue if eaten in excess. There is a higher omega 3 content and quality protein. They have no antibiotics, pesticides, steroids, dyes, and are low in PCB (polychlorinated biphenyls), which are chlorine atoms that come from food manufacturers. PCB are toxins produced from waste in industrial processing.

Farm Raised Fish

1. Enclosed cage	5. Less quality protein
2. Less exercise	6. Higher diseased prone
3. Antibiotics, steroids	7. Higher toxins, fat, xenoestrogens
4. Artificially colored	

Farm raised fish are enclosed inside cages in lakes, ponds, rivers or oceans. The fish get less exercise, and less nutritious foods and they live and swim in their waste. This fish has been discovered to be treated with antibiotics and steroids, including being artificially colored, having low quality protein, more contaminates, higher fat content, lower omega 3, prone to higher mercury and high Xenoestrogen PCB (Polychlorinated Biphenyls).

Free Radicals vs. Super Antioxidants

Health and healing begin at the cellular level - from the inside out! Free radicals inflame the body and make the body's ecosystem unstable. They have been linked to DNA damages, accelerated aging, the breakdown of organs, and premature cellular death. They are called "free radicals" because they have no charge in them and need one or more charges to become stable. So, they float around looking to become stable with an electron charge. Human living cells have the electrons they want. So living cell are a target.

Through an oxidation process, free radicals steal living cells' electrons. This leaves the living cells without their paired electrons to function and survive, which in turn makes them unstable themselves. Then they turn into free radicals themselves, seeking a paired electron from other living cells. They rob Peter to pay Paul, and a chain reaction occurs which is dangerous if not stopped.

A researcher and Professor, Jeffrey Blumberg of Tufts University in Medford, Massachusetts said that free radicals are dangerous because they don't just damage one molecule of a cell, but one free radical can set off a whole chain reaction across many cells. It does that by oxidizing a fatty acid and changes that fatty acid into a free radical itself. It's a very rapid chain reaction. However, there is help.

King Antioxidants To The Rescue!
Naturally, the human body can make its own free radicals to destroy detrimental bacteria or viruses. But the body uses special enzymes to break those free radicals down and then get rid of them. They do that to help keep human cells from further harm. Antioxidant nutrients help the body by donating their own electrons to satisfy the free radical unpaired electrons. This saves human living cells from destruction. Antioxidants are powerful nutrients that not only fight for the body, but at the same time strengthen our body. What a marvelous plan!

Free radicals are in non-food-based chemicals, such as environmental toxic chemicals, radiation, cigarette smoke, pesticides, pollution, vehicle exhaust, and industrial and household cleaning chemicals. We get Antioxidants from dietary sources, such as, fruits, vegetables, grains, nuts, beans and sufficiently from herbs.

High Antioxidant Foods

Herbs and Spices are #1 scavengers of free radicals. Most nutritionists recommend eating 5-8 servings of fruits and vegetables per day. This can help protect the body from ramped free radicals from taking over the cells. This will also help the immune system become stronger or more resilient, especially those that suffer with weak immunity, like babies, children, pregnant mothers and the elderly.

Super sources of antioxidants are the following.

1. Fruits and vegetables	7. Green teas (flavonoids)
2. Vitamin E (tocopherols)	8. Melatonin, selenium and zinc
3. Vitamin A (beta-carotene)	9. Multivitamin, (are a mix of vitamins, minerals and amino acids)
4. Vitamin C	
5. CoQ10	
6. Quercetin	

ORAC

ORAC stands for Oxygen Radical Absorbance Capacity. It is a measure of the ability of a food to quench the oxygenation of free radicals. The measuring's of the antioxidant absorbent capacity of free radicals was developed by the National Institute on Aging, which is also the National Institutes of Health. For example, here is a list of ORAC values of spices and foods.

1. Sumac, bran, raw 312,400 ORAC
2. Spices, cloves, ground 290,283 ORAC
3. Sorghum, bran, hi-tannin 240,000 ORAC
4. Oregano, dried 175,295 ORAC
5. Rosemary, dried 165,280 ORAC
6. Thyme, dried 157,380 ORAC
7. Cinnamon, ground 131,420 ORAC
8. Spices, turmeric, ground 127,068 ORAC
9. Sorghum, bran, red 71,000 ORAC
10. Nutmeg, ground 69,640 ORAC
11. Basil, dried 61,063 ORAC
12. Cocoa, dry powder, unsweet 55,653 ORAC
13. Raspberries, black 19,220 ORAC
14. Nuts, walnuts, English 13,541 ORAC
15. Juice, black raspberry 10,460 ORAC
16. Vanilla beans, dry 122,400 ORAC
17. Sage, ground 119,929 ORAC
18. Spice, szechuan pepper, 118,400 ORAC
19. Acai, fruit pulp/skin, powder. 102,700 ORAC
20. Sorghum, bran, black 100,800 ORAC

21. Rosehip 96,150 ORAC
22. Sumac, grain, raw 86,800 ORAC
23. Spices, parsley, dried 73,670 ORAC
24. Raisins, golden seedless 10,450 ORAC
25. Nuts, hazelnuts or filberts 9,645 ORAC
26. Blueberries, wild, raw 9,621 ORAC
27. Pears, dried (Italy) 9,496 ORAC
28. Savory, fresh 9,465 ORAC
29. Cranberries, raw 9,090 ORAC
30. Artichokes, Ocean Mist, boiled 9,416 ORAC
31. Beans, kidney, red, raw 8,606 ORAC
32. Beans, black, raw 8,494 ORAC
33. Beans, pinto, raw 8,033 ORAC
34. Currants, European black, raw 7,957 ORAC
35. Pistachio nuts, raw 7,675 ORAC
36. Plums, black diamond, raw 7,581 ORAC
37. Agave, dried (Southwest) 7,524 ORAC
38. Candies, milk chocolate 7,519 ORAC
39. Blackberries, raw 5,905 ORAC
40. Garlic powder 6,665 ORAC
41. Chocolate syrup, non-sweet 6,330 ORAC
42. Plums, raw 6,100 ORAC
43. Artichokes, (globe/French), raw 6,552 ORAC
44. Baby food, peaches 6,257 ORAC

12 Water Demands Of The Body

It is said, a person cannot live past 3-4 days without water. Water helps the body in many ways. It's needed among other things for processing and manufacturing nutrients for the body. Among other good things, cellular fluids are made with water. Water carries oxygen to cells, tissues and organs, and also hydrates, detoxifies, used for energy and fat. It removes toxins and waste from the body too. The human body carries between 65% - 75% water.

1. The brain requires up to 75%.
2. It constitutes 22% of the bones, 75% of muscles, 65-85% cartilage, and 83% of cellular fluids.
3. Cushions joints and required for flexibility.
4. It helps the liver filter toxins and helps it make specific nutrients to feed the body.
5. It helps digestion in nutrient assimilation and absorption.
6. It helps carry nutrients to organ systems.
7. It helps the spleen process white and red blood cells.
8. It helps the gallbladder for its bile maintenance and flushes excess cholesterol.

9. It moistens and hydrates the lungs for oxygen utilization.
10. It facilitates the removal of waste in all areas of the body.
11. It moistens the colon for bowel regularity and assist in the removal of waste and toxins.
12. It is required by the kidneys to regulate the body's fluid balance, including blood pressure.

Types Of Drinking Water

Now I'm going to talk about drinking water to give you some insight on how they are processed so you can make the best decision for yourself and family.

1. Tap water	6. Distilled
2. Surface	7. Reverse osmosis
3. Ground	8. Sparkling water
4. Artesian	9. Home water purification system
5. Deionized	

Surface Water (Tap)

1. Spring water	4. Collected in reservoirs

| 2. Lakes, streams and creeks
3. Self-purified | 5. 100% purified bottled water |

Surface water is above the ground and comes from lakes, streams and creeks. Tap water comes from this water either from a private well or public municipal water treatment system. It's collected in reservoirs and piped into the faucets of homes. We cook, drink, wash, and flush our commodes with surface water.

Surface water is spring water. 100% spring bottled water must be pure, and the label must list the spring where the water came from. Surface water purifies itself by running over rocks and exchanging its impurities for the rock's minerals, which then turns it into spring mineral water. Carbon gas is added to bottled spring water. This is how it gets its fizz.

Depending on the county you live in will determine if your water is surface or ground water.

Surface water is the easiest contaminated by environmental chemical toxins by rainwater runoff from businesses, homes, parking lots and roads. The chemical company DuPoint®

polluted county waters. They were sued by residents in 2006 for polluting the water supply in Salem County, New Jersey with a carcinogen perfluorooctanoic (PFOA) used for the production of Teflon. They settled in 2011 for $8.3 million. DuPont® was also sued in 2004, by Ohio, West Virginia residents. They settled for $343 million, and gave $70 million in medical evaluations for the residents.

Ground Water (Tap)

Ground water flows from beneath the ground's surface and then flows into a water table system and transfers to the surface and then gets extracted through wells. Well water has better minerals, but then there is a higher risk of toxin contamination because it naturally mixes with surface water. However, impurities are removed commercially.

Ground water is filtered to remove bacteria, viruses, parasites, pesticides, fertilizers, asbestos, drugs, and heavy metals, like; radon, arsenic, aluminum, lead and others. Therefore, purification systems can be excellent, but some impurities can still remain in both ground and surface water.

Manufacturers do disinfect it with fluorine and chlorine. Other chemicals may be added to make the water clearer or taste better. Have you ever drunk Tap Water and it taste like chlorine?

Well water can be collected in reservoirs like surface or spring water. It is piped into homes and businesses and used for watering the grass, cooking, drinking, bathing, washing clothes and dishes, including flushing commodes.

For more information about the quality and type of tap water that comes out of your faucets, visit EPA.gov to see your county and your subdivision's water source.

Ground Water (Artesian)

1. Deeper below	5. Minimal Contamination
2. By Pressure	
3. Protected	6. Mineral-based
4. Bottled Water	

Artesian water is deep below the surface and naturally flows to the surface by pressure. It passes into wells, and then commercial companies process and purify it. Artesian water is enclosed by rocks and protected by the layers of pores in the rocks. It is less likely contaminated than surface water, and has higher mineral contents. It's found in bottled drinking water.

Distilled (Spring Water)

1. CPAP Machine 2. Steamed 3. Impurities removed	4. Not as pure as Deionized water 5. Bottled water

Distilled water can be both from ground or spring. Manufacturers process it by steam. This steam water has a heavier taste, but it's a good option with the minerals and impurities removed. However, deionized water is purer.

Distilled water is good for CPAP machines because when the water evaporates, there are few minerals to interact with oxygen and may not dry-out the mouth.

Reverse Osmosis

1. Ground or spring 2. CPAP machines	4. Impurities removed

| 3. Better | 5. Bottled water |

It can be both from ground or spring water, and it is ideal for CPAP machines. Reverse osmosis filtration removes minerals and impurities by way of a steam process. Manufacturers boil the water and let it evaporate. Then the steam is collected after bacteria, viruses, chemicals, pollutants and minerals fall to the bottom in a separate tank where they are discarded. We can cook and eat with this water. It is a better choice of water for the sick because of its low impurities. Minerals can be replaced with a good vegetable juice or fresh lemon water.

Sparkling Water

| 1. Ground or spring
2. Oxygen and carbon | 3. Dissolves under pressure
4. Bottled water |

I make my own soda pop by mixing sparkling water with my favorite fruit juice. Sparkling can be both from ground or spring. It is a mix of carbon and oxygen, where the carbon dioxide gas dissolves in the water under pressure. We see carbonated bottled drinking water at stores.

An example of sparkling water is the green bottle Perrier® from France, which is my favorite sparkling water beverage. It's better than soda pop. I began drinking Perrier® when I was in Europe – Sofia, Bulgaria, which is a 3 to 9-hour drive from Thessaloniki, Macedonia, Philippi, Corinth and Athens. By the way, I like Mediterranean food. When I was there, I found the food good for my health. I give it a scale of 1-10 where 10 being the highest quality.

In Sofia, Bulgaria, they don't use the amounts of synthetic chemicals, pesticides, and hydrogenated, rancid oils like the USA. The food is preserved naturally. I was not sick. It actually made my skin, hair, nails, lungs, even my eye sight better. To my surprise, I did not use as many dietary supplements when I was there. However, I was prepared and brought my first aid concoctions just in case I needed to kill parasites, heal wounds, stop bleeding or food poisoning.

Home Water Purification System

1. For showers 2. For kitchen faucets	4. Sold at Lowes 5. Bed Bath and Beyond®

| 3. Sold at Home Depot® | 6. Sold at grocery stores |

It's a good idea for everyone to have a water purification system in their home, especially if living in the city or near a mining or chemical processing plant. Water purification systems can help remove water impurities like drug residues, heavy metals, viruses and environmental chemicals. Keep in mind that if you install a whole-house water purification system, then you will not need to install individuals on your shower heads or kitchen sink faucets.

Food Combining for Easier Digestion

Our body functioning's are very organized. Good digestion and absorption is everything in the recovery process. It is not hard to bring digestion into good balance. It may happen sooner rather than later when it's given what it needs to improve.

Contrary to popular belief, you are not what you eat. You are what you only absorb into your organs, tissues and cells. It's the nutritious nutrients that give the body vitality and life, while excess junk foods, toxins and emotional stress tend to weaken the body and set the stage for disease.

When stomach acid, digestion and assimilation of nutrients are off balance, organs tend to become stressed, undernourished and irritable like little babies. They need their food supply to survive. But if not, symptoms tend to appear on the scene. The body communicates with signals (nerves) warning us of approaching health problems. Digestive juices in proper balance is key when breaking food down. When the digestive tract is improved and strengthened naturally, symptoms will be easier to address everywhere in the body.

3 Basic Guidelines For Digestion

1. Rule 1	Not combining proteins and starches together.
2. Rule 2	Not combining fruit and melons together.
3. Rule 3	Chewing food at least 27 times until its liquified. It helps the digestive track digest the food easier, and make it ready for assimilation into organs, tissues and cells.

It's healthier allowing proper time for food to digest before changing food categories because it may reduce the risk of foods fermenting in the gut. For example, the fruit will digest and ferment in the gut before meat finishes digesting first. See the chart below.

Typical Food Digestion Before Assimilation

12 Hours	Meats
5 Hours	Vegetables (and starches), Beans, Eggs, Milk, Protein Drinks, Nuts and Cheeses
2 Hours	Fruits
1 Hour	Melons
30 Minutes	Fruit / Vegetable Juices

Acidosis And Alkalosis

It is well known that symptoms can arise in the body from a pH imbalance of over acidity or over alkalinity. Too much acids in the body and not enough alkalinity to neutralize that acid can becomes a problem, and vs. versa with too much alkalinity and not enough acidity in the body.

Armor of God

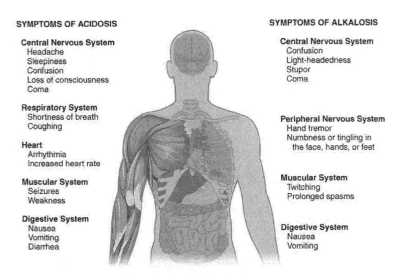

SYMPTOMS OF ACIDOSIS

Central Nervous System
Headache
Sleepiness
Confusion
Loss of consciousness
Coma

Respiratory System
Shortness of breath
Coughing

Heart
Arrhythmia
Increased heart rate

Muscular System
Seizures
Weakness

Digestive System
Nausea
Vomiting
Diarrhea

SYMPTOMS OF ALKALOSIS

Central Nervous System
Confusion
Light-headedness
Stupor
Coma

Peripheral Nervous System
Hand tremor
Numbness or tingling in the face, hands, or feet

Muscular System
Twitching
Prolonged spasms

Digestive System
Nausea
Vomiting

Source: Anatomy & Physiology, Connexions Web site. cnx.org/content/col11496/1.6/, Jun 19, 2013. Author: OpenStax College

The upper stomach has 4.0 - 6.5 pH (acidic). The lower stomach has 1.5 - 4.0 pH (acidic). The duodenum, which is the first part of the small intestines has a 7.0 - 8.5 pH (neutral to alkaline). It's there that the pancreas releases enzymes to break down protein, carbs and fats. It also releases sodium bicarbonate to neutralize the acid before passing it into the rest of the small intestines, which is 4.0 - 7.0 pH - acidic to neutral.

The sodium bicarbonate helps reduce the lower stomach acid from burning holes in sensitive duodenum tissues. Otherwise, there would be a potential for peptic ulcer formations and H. Pylori proliferation.

When the duodenum task is complete, it releases the nutrients into the rest of the small intestines to be absorbed by the bloodstream. This is an important process because the acids have to be neutralized before the nutrients can be absorbed into the bloodstream. Otherwise, the whole body would be challenged with an off balance homeostatis.

Blood is 7.4 pH, Saliva pH is 6.5 - 7.5, and Urine is 4.5 - 8 pH, (the ideal is 6 - 7.4 pH).

On average in an adult, it takes 256 ounces of pure water for organs to overcome the acid in an 8 ounce can of soda pop. That's 1 soda pop and 32 cups of water to overcome the acid. Coffee is more than that. You can see that one can of soda pop can require a lot more effort to counterbalance the acid. Lower stomach acid pH is 1.5 - 4.0. See the below chat. Note: Lemons, orange juice, grapefruit juice and vinegar (except raw apple cider vinegar, have an alkaline effect after digestion. But starts off acidic at first.

pH in These Foods, including Battery Acid

• Tap water 7.7 – 7.0
• Cow's Milk
  6.4 – 6.8
• Cheddar cheese
  5.9 – 6.0
• Bread
  5.0 – 6.2
• Root beer
  3.8 – 4.0
• Honey
  3.7 – 4.2
• Orange juice*
  3.3 – 4.2
• Diet cola
  3.0 – 3.3
	• Grapefruit*
	  3.0 – 3.8
	• Vinegar*
	  2.4 – 3.4
	• Coffee
	  2.4 – 3.3
	• Cola
	  2.4 – 2.5
	• Sports drinks
	  2.3 – 4.4
	• Wine
	  2.3 – 3.8
	• Lemon juice*
	  2.0 – 2.6
	• Battery acid
	  1.0

Armor of God

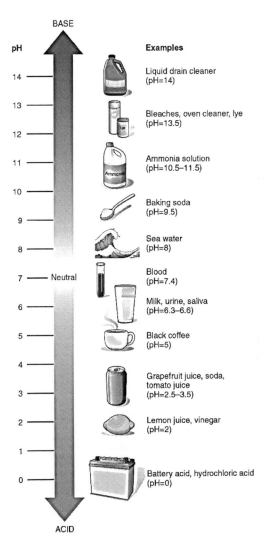

Source: Anatomy & Physiology, Connexions Web site. cnx.org/content/col11496/1.6/, Jun 19, 2013. Author: OpenStax College

A pH Test Strip measures the alkalinity and acidity of the fluids in the body. It gives a metric of the environment that organs are adapting in.

1. The Saliva pH tests reveal the level of alkalinity of organ mineral reserves and indicates how well nutrients are being absorbed from foods into the body's organs, tissues and cells.
2. The Urine pH test measures the metrics of how well the kidneys are buffering extracellular fluid acids. The lower the number the more acidic it is. The higher the number, the more alkaline it is. It's the midpoint where the body naturally needs to be.

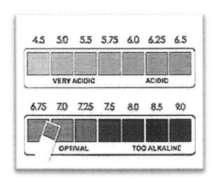

Some people are more alkaline than they are acidic, or vs. versa. In other words, does everyone need an alkaline diet? It doesn't appear that way if they are over alkaline already. An acidic diet can help balance out the alkalinity. See the chart on Acidosis and Alkalosis.

If blood pH is too acidic, it can put organs at risk of damage. That's why balancing the pH is important for wellness and recovery.

Think of the stomach as a fireplace. When it burns food down, the food turns into an ash. The ash is the nutrients that were removed from the food. This ash is going to be absorbed by the bloodstream and carried to organs, tissues and cells; however, the pH balance of stomach acid has to be right for this to take place properly.

Acidic Foods

The following foods are acidic - below 7 pH.

Note, * These foods leave an alkaline ash in the body, but have an acidifying effect after digestion.

Apples*, Bacon, Barley, Beef, Blueberries*, Bran Oat, Bread (white), Bread (whole wheat), Butter, Carob, Cheese, Chicken, Codfish, Corn, Corned beef, Crackers (soda), Cranberries,* Eggs, Flour (white), Flour (whole wheat), Haddock, Honey, Lamb, Lentils, Plums* Lobster, Milk (cow's), Macaroni, Oatmeal, Oysters, Peanut Butter, Peas (dried), Pike, Pork, Prunes*, Rice (brown and white), Salmon, Sardines, Sausage, Scallops, Shrimps, Spaghetti, Squash, Winter, Sunflower seeds, Turkey, Veal, Walnuts, Wheat germ, and Yogurt.

Alkaline Foods

The following list of alkaline foods are at or above a 7 pH.

They help balance the body's pH so acidic compounds do not weaken organs. Alkaline foods are vegetables, most fruits and almonds. Most organs are made of alkalinity, except the upper stomach. Some alkaline minerals are potassium, magnesium, and zinc.

Almonds, Apples, Apricots, Avocados, Bananas, Beans, dried, Beet Greens, Beets, Blackberries, Broccoli, Brussels sprouts, Cabbage,

Carrots, Cauliflower, Celery, Chard Leaves, Cherries (sour), Cucumber, Dates (dried), Figs (dried), Grapefruit, Grapes, Green beans, Green peas, Green Rutabagas, Lemons, Lettuce, Lima beans, Limes, Milk-goat's* Millet, Molasses, Mushrooms, Muskmelon, Onions, Oranges, Parsnip, Peaches, Pears, Pineapple, Potatoes (sweet), Potatoes (white), Radishes, Raisins, Raspberries, Sauerkraut, Spinach (raw), Strawberries, Tangerines, Tomatoes, Watercress, and Watermelon.

Oral Health: Fighting Infections

Water-Pik, Toothpaste, Toothbrush, Hydrogen peroxide and Dental floss. These are time tested solutions that have helped keep bacteria from infecting the gums and teeth.

Getting under the gums is crucial for uprooting disease creating microorganisms. Unfortunately, traditional toothbrushes are not ideal for washing harmful bacteria from under the gums, but a Waterpik can get in there and do a very good job. A Waterpik is a "Water Flosser." Dentist are known to use them. For sensitive teeth, the water flosser's pressure can be adjusted to a comfortable level.

After a while, Toothbrushes accumulate bacteria, so to kill bacteria, we spray inside the mouth a small amount of hydrogen peroxide and water, then gargle and spit it out. This combination has worked wonderfully throughout history for neutralizing or killing germs and limiting plaque buildup. We also rinse the mouth a second time with water only and then spit it out, and then brush our teeth and rinse and spit that out too 😊 We are thorough because we try to avoid going to the doctors and accumulating medical bills. We also replace toothbrushes every summer, fall, winter, and spring.

Natural toothpaste can be made with a little baking soda, a drop of tea tree oil and or peppermint oil. Those oils automatically freshen the breath. They can be found in toothpastes. Some people like Listerine, but the dye-free one is a better choice in that case.

Most traditional Toothpaste ingredients have a detergent in them called Sodium Lauryl Sulfate (SLS). This is toxic to health. The back of a box of detergent says to call poison control if the detergent is swallowed. SLS is used in shampoos, hair conditioners, laundry soap and dish detergent products. SLS separates molecules so that the interaction between the product and the teeth can work better.

Natural toothpaste is healthier for the body because they're normally free from toxic chemicals, artificial colors, flavorings and preservatives. But still no guarantee because of changing regulations. They can't guarantee cavity reduction either because that all depends on how well the teeth are taken care of. Excessive toxins, sugar, coffee, soda pop, and alcoholic beverages can decay teeth quicker. However, the teeth and gums still can balance themselves when given what they need to heal.

Importance Of Natural Deodorant

Aluminum is the main ingredient in traditional deodorants. When excessive amounts of this metal are used, it finds its way into the bloodstream and soft tissues of the body. It may then slow metabolic activities and delay the healing process.

When skin pores are blocked-up with waste – old debris, it makes it harder for the bloodstream to release waste from there.

High aluminum has the potential to hinder blood vessels from absorbing water and other minerals too. Good nutrients are essential for the body in gaining strength to release waste. It takes energy. Lymph nodes are positioned at the armpits as well as throughout the body. Armpits should never be blocked by aluminum all day long, especially while sleeping.

Traditional aluminum deodorants usually have 18-25% aluminum, but aluminum free deodorants have none. It's easy to mask scent by using an essential oil with the aluminum free deodorant. Some good essential oils for males are cedarwood, myrrh or sage. For females, peppermint, rose, grapefruit, or lavender smells nice. To reduce or stop skin irritation, essential oils can be diluted with castor oil, olive oil or another light edible oil.

Importance Of Natural Menstrual Products

The best ones are organic, 100% cotton with no bleach (chlorine), no chemical dyes, no fragrances, and no plastic materials. Washable pads are also available.

Most traditional female hygiene products are bleached with chlorine, dyed, and scented with artificial perfumes. These toxic chemicals have the potential to generate free radicals and put stress on the organs. When buying panty-liners, pads, or tampons, it's ideal to look for ones that are not dyed, bleached, perfumed, or have artificial chemicals or plastic. However, most tampons have a warning label of "toxic shock", therefore not a good choice and should be avoided.

Using tampons regularly increases a woman's risk towards uterine health problems. Traditional ones have artificial and toxic chemicals which can absorb into the bloodstream and spread to the lymph nodes and disrupt the natural balance of the uterus. If you use Tampons, the better choice is choosing all natural.

BONUS DEVOTIONAL

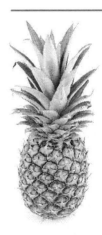

Do not forsake her (wisdom), and she will preserve you; Love her, and she will keep you. Wisdom is the principal thing; Therefore get wisdom. And in all your getting, get understanding. Proverbs 4:6-7

Times Up Devil – Get Thee Behind Me!
Day 1: Know Your Real Enemy

Be sober, be vigilant; because your adversary the devil, as a roaring lion, walketh about, seeking whom he may devour.
1 Peter 5:8

When you hear the word "enemy," you may think about someone who has wronged you, or, you may think about bad people in the world who seek to cause harm.

But the Bible is clear about who our real enemy is. Satan is not only like a roaring lion, seeking whom he may devour, he is also the father of all lies. From the moment he was cast out of heaven, he has been roaming the earth trying to deceive as many people as possible.

Satan and his demon have used opioids as a stronghold tactic to entangle, steal, kill, and destroy millions of people. He is the adversary of your soul. When we recognize the true source of our battle, we can then arm ourselves with the exact thing that combats him better than anything else can.

The Word of God, in the name of Jesus, will overcome Satan at every turn. By arming yourself with Scriptures to throw in the face of the enemy, he will have no choice but to flee. Try a few of these passages the next time Satan comes around:

Thanks be to God, who gives us the victory through our Lord Jesus Christ. 1 Corinthians 15:57

'Not by might nor by power, but by My Spirit,' says the Lord of hosts. Zechariah 4:6

The Lord will cause your enemies who rise against you to be defeated before your face; they shall come out against you one way and flee before you seven ways. Deuteronomy 28:7

❖ Say and write these words 3 times: "The Lord Jesus Christ Rebuke you Satan! Get thee behind me. You shall serve the Lord thy God and He only shall you serve. Amen!"

Prayer Journal:

Day 2: Don't Believe Lies Of The Enemy

Again, the devil taketh Him up into an exceeding high mountain, and sheweth Him all the kingdoms of the world, and the glory of them; and saith unto Him, "All these things will I give Thee, if Thou wilt fall down and worship me."
Matthew 4:8-9

The lies of the enemy come in all shapes and sizes. From the smallest deception to the biggest ploy, his assaults are endless towards the people of God. And if the devil can wear us down, he can weaken us to the point where we begin to believe his lies.

So, how can we decipher the lies of the enemy? Anytime the truth is twisted, the works of Satan is behind it. He has mastered how to make something seem true but twist it in his favor to get men to fail. It takes a steadfast knowledge of the Word of God through scripture and faith to expose the lies of the devil.

Just before Jesus' ministry on earth, He was led by the Holy Spirit into the desert where He fasted and prayed. During His forty days, He was tired and hungry, and in His vulnerability, Satan showed up to tempt Him. But Jesus was more than ready to combat the lies with Scripture. He simply quoted the words of the Scriptures in answer to the enemy's deceptions.

I love this account in the Bible because it shows Jesus' humanity and His Lordship. For He was at his lowest point physically, but at His strongest Spiritually. Why? Because He had spent time alone with the Father, praying, fasting, and meditating on the Word.

That is KEY to recognizing and overcoming the lies of the enemy. We must get alone with God and devote ample time to prayer and study of the Word. Then, when the enemy comes prowling, we will have the exact answers to get rid of him in a hurry.

❖ Look at your calendar and find a time when you can get away for at least a day and a night. Remove yourself from the day-to-day schedule and take that time to fast, pray, and read the Scriptures. Arm yourself with fool-proof words from the Scriptures to combat the enemy's lies.

Prayer Journal:

_____
_____
_____
_____
_____
_____
_____
_____
_____
_____
_____
_____
_____
_____
_____
_____
_____
_____
_____
_____
_____
_____
_____
_____
_____

Day 3: Illness: Satan's Advantage

*Heal me, O Lord, and I shall be healed;
save me, and I shall be saved:
for Thou art my praise.
Jeremiah 17:14*

Leave it to the enemy to kick us when we are down. It doesn't take much for Satan to recognize an opportunity to tempt us in our weakness. Especially when we have committed ourselves to Jesus Christ, Satan's aim is to take away our strength and vitality by inflicting weakness and sickness.

But God...

God is the Great Healer, Protector, and Defender. He will fight for us when we cannot. He will be a shield around us and a strong tower of refuge. We need only to lift hands of praise in the midst of illness, and call upon Jesus Christ to heal and defend. If we do that, Satan doesn't stand a chance no matter what the circumstance.

Be vigilant, don't allow Satan to get the upper hand during times of illness. Fight back with praise, worship, and full dependence on God to make you well. Illness does not have to be a time of defeat, but a time of refreshing and complete rest in the Lord's defense.

If you are battling illness, allow yourself to fully rest in the Lord's provision. Use this time to pray, worship, and read the Scriptures. When the enemy tries to take advantage of your weakness, call out to God and rebuke Satan in Jesus name. For when we are weak, Jesus is very strong.

- ❖ Write down what you have been struggling with and then write over it "I AM STRONGER - JESUS IS MY ROCK!"

Prayer Journal:

_____
_____
_____
_____

Armor of God

Day 4: The Accuser

Then I heard a loud voice saying in heaven, "Now salvation, and strength, and the kingdom of our God, and the power of His Christ have come, for the accuser of our brethren, who accused them before our God day and night, has been cast down.
Revelation 12:10

Nothing holds us back from living a victorious life more than guilt or shame. Past and present faults hover in our minds and often keep us from stepping out in faith.

The accuser of our souls—Satan—will always be there to whisper words of condemnation. He aims to never let us forget our trespasses. And if he can get us to remember our guilt, he will keep us from living in the freedom of the Holy Spirit.

For where the Spirit of the Lord is, there is freedom. 2 Corinthians 3:17

One of Satan's tactics is condemnation, guilt and shame. Declare, today, that your accuser has no more power over you. Take a stand against Satan and his lies. Face every whisper of condemnation with shouts of truth from God's Word. The blood of the Lamb has defeated the accuser!

All authority is Christ's, and He has taken every sin and shame and nailed it to the cross once and for all. Do not let the accuser deceive you any longer. Cling to the old rugged cross and the ultimate sacrifice Jesus paid. For He paid ALL for you.

- ❖ Today, make a list of all the things that hold you back from living in freedom. Present that list to the Lord and declare that Jesus Christ has wiped the slate clean. Then, write over it. "I AM FREE IN JESUS NAME."

Prayer Journal:

_____
_____
_____
_____
_____

Armor of God

Day 5: Wrong Pride: Satan's Tactics

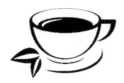

Humble yourselves in the sight of the Lord, and He shall lift you up.
James 4:10

There is a reason why the Scriptures tell us that pride comes before a fall. The wrong pride keeps our hearts elevated on "self" instead of fixated on God. It keeps our heads held high—so high, we aren't watching where we are going. And before long, the enemy places something in front of us to trip us up.

Satan will always use pride to turn our focus from the Holy Spirit and onto our own abilities. And, as we all know, our own abilities don't get us very far. Will-power always runs out of power sooner or later. That is why the Bible states, *"not by power nor by might, but by my Spirit, says the Lord."* Zechariah 4:6

Let's not give Satan a foothold by allowing pride to enter our minds and hearts. With every thought of self-centeredness or self-reliance, let us humble ourselves before the mighty hand of God and know that He will lift us up in due time.

Be watchful of where you are going. The enemy is waiting on the sidelines to trip you up at any moment. There is no room for pride in the heart of the believer. For God is our strength and provision.

❖ If you struggle with pride, take a few moments to get alone with God and confess it today. Humble yourself before the Lord and ask Him for a heart of humility. Satan can't do anything with a humble and contrite heart.

Prayer Journal:

_____
_____
_____
_____
_____
_____
_____
_____

Armor of God

Matters Of The Heart: Breaking Strongholds.
Day 6: Unresolved Unforgiveness

Shouldest not thou also have had compassion on thy fellow servant,
even as I had pity on thee?
Matthew 18:33

Jesus lovingly, yet firmly, taught his disciples in the form of parables. To get His point across, He used examples that they would relate to and easily understand. It was important to Him that they grasped the principal meaning of what He was trying to teach them.

That parable of the unforgiving servant was such a story – See Matthew 23-35. In it, Jesus described a king who demanded that one of his servants pay an outstanding debt. When the servant could not, the king ordered him and his family to be sold to pay the debt instead. The servant, however, pleaded for mercy, and the king had compassion on him, forgiving his debt and sending him on his way. Instead of going on his way rejoicing at the king's mercy, the servant went out and found someone who owed him money and forcefully ordered him to repay it. When the person could not, he had him thrown into prison. When the king heard about it, he handed him over to be tortured in prison.

Truly, this is a clear picture of unforgiveness.

We, too, have been forgiven of every sin and shame through Christ Jesus our Lord, yet we struggle to extend it to others. Unresolved unforgiveness only opens doors of torture into our lives – whether it be mentally, physically or spiritually. It deepens our wounds and prevents the healing we so desperately need.

Will you choose to forgive someone today? Do you want peace, joy, and happiness? It's your right. You can have it and claim that peace in your life.

- ❖ Write a letter or an email to someone who has offended you. Be honest with them about the pain they have caused but release the unforgiveness once and for all.

Allow the Lord to bring you sweet healing and deliverance. Your soul could be thirsting for it.

- ❖ If the person is not available, no problem! Just journal your thoughts below and release the unforgiveness. If you must cry or scream to get it out, then let it out now. Shout seven times "Jesus" until that unforgiveness lose its grip on you.

Prayer Journal:

_____
_____
_____
_____
_____
_____
_____
_____
_____
_____
_____
_____
_____
_____
_____

Armor of God

Day 7: Unresolved Anger and Bitterness

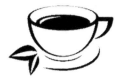

Follow peace with all men, and holiness, without which no man shall see the Lord: looking diligently lest any man fail of the grace of God; lest any root of bitterness springing up trouble you, and thereby many be defiled.
Hebrews 12:14-15

Unresolved anger is a troublesome thing. It sets us on edge, steals our joy, and corrupts our lives with bitterness.

The Bible says that once bitterness takes root, trouble will spring up. It will cause all sorts of unloving reactions. Eventually, it will cause us to act upon those impulses and lead us into a life of compromise.

What is at the heart of our anger? When we really stop to think about it, what causes us to react angrily instead of responding lovingly?

For some of us, we need to go way back in time, to that first dangerous spark of anger. We need to confront the hurts that eventually led to unresolved anger and bitterness. Only then, will we be able to recognize what sets us off today. Only then, will we be able to stop our outbursts and reactive anger.

Seeking peace and holiness with all men is the solution that Hebrews 12:14 gives us. It is the deliberate act of making amends with those who have angered us and coming to terms by releasing things that have formed bitterness within us.

Only then, will we be able to clearly see the grace of God and walk in it.

❖ On the side, jot down trivial things that make you angry. (kids leaving socks on the floor, impatient drivers, and so on). Then, on the right side, write your deep-seeded angers. (being unappreciated, misunderstood, lied to, taken advantage of, mistreated, and so on). See the difference? Tackle the root issues of anger and allow God's love to free you from its grasp!

Trivial Things	Deep-Seated Anger

Day 8: Unresolved Hurts

Terrors are turned upon me: they pursue my soul as the wind: and my welfare passeth away as a cloud. And now my soul is poured out upon me; the days of affliction have taken hold upon me.
Job 30:15-16

This type of hurt is an emotional pain. Although it is not a physical pain, it is a soul pain that will stimulate a delayed or sudden physical manifestation of symptoms. In my practice, I have seen muscle tremors, nausea, migraine headaches, nervous fatigue and stress to name a few. I've seen symptoms resolved after hurts were identified and the Lord touched their heart. Plus, a custom diet plan and dietary supplements to replenish the nutrients the body used-up to for fighting the stress.

Perhaps, no one in all of history experienced hurt quite like Job. This man's unimaginable pain was recorded in the Old Testament as a testimony of unwavering faith and ultimate healing through the mighty hand of God.

What deep hurts remain as tormentors in your soul? What past offenses are keeping God's healing touch at arm's Program Length? It is time to come face-to-face with unresolved hurts. Now, more than ever before, the victory can be yours.

Jesus Himself was wounded for those very things that hurt you in the first place. He took on every insult people threw your way. Then He nailed those hurts to a wooden cross – for good.

❖ Take a walk in the sunshine with your favorite worship song. Keep in step to the music as you allow the Holy Spirit's comfort to wash over and in you. Journal below and release all hurts, past and present to Him and rejoice in your deliverance. Surender all control and finally breathe deep and let it go!

_____
_____
_____
_____

Armor of God

Day 9: Abandonment

Hide not Thy face far from me; put not
Thy servant away in anger: Thou hast
been my help; leave me not, neither forsake
me, O God of my salvation. When my
father and my mother forsake me,
then the Lord will take me up.
Psalm 27:9-10

Alone…

That's how we feel in the depths of our addictions. We believe that no one else understands the despair we feel. And those feelings only cast us further into the depths of addiction's grip.

Take heart! Look up! There is One who knows! He has not forsaken you. He has not abandoned you. In fact, right now, He is drawing you near. He is welcoming you into His everlasting arms.

Do you feel it? Do you feel HIM? Call His name! The Almighty God of the Universe is inviting you to reside in Him forever!

All the lost years of abandonment are reconciled in Christ Jesus. Every tear that has fallen has fallen at the feet of a tender and compassionate King.

You are not alone.

*Today, contact 2-3 trusted people and invite them to be part of your prayer team. Make this team of people your go-to group who will pray for you any time of the day or night. The truth is, we need God and we need each other. Don't walk this journey alone. Who do you want to call? The 700 Club is available also 1-800-700-7000.

_____
_____
_____
_____
_____
_____
_____
_____

Day 10: Soul, Emotional-Ties vs. Agape Love

Do not be unequally yoked together with unbelievers. For what fellowship has righteousness with lawlessness? And what communion has light with darkness?
2 Corinthians 6:14

Nothing that we do on this earth is purely physical. Because we are made up of body, mind, spirit and soul, everything we experience engages all four facets (sides) of our being.

We would like to believe that we can separate our emotions from our bodies, or our minds from our souls, but we simply cannot. We need to view each of our actions in the light of how we were created.

Soul-ties are strong-bonds that form by the act of sexual contact - sex outside of marriage or within marriage. Multiple partners lead to multiple Soul-Ties and this can lead to marriage challenges due to the multiple Soul-Tie influences. God must be allowed to separate past Soul-Ties from the marriage-bond in order for the marriage to have better peace.

Emotional-Ties are formed through friendships that have no sexual relationship. Some Emotional-Ties can be a heavy weight on the other person. It's like a co-dependence. The person who is chronically injecting their emotions, stress and life challenges becomes the other person's life. Then these things influence that person's life and choices. These types of heavy Emotional-Ties need to be cut off so that a person can heal and make progress in their life. For example, if the person is always feeling stuck or unsuccessful, then this may be one of the underlying root problems interfering. Heavy Emotional-Ties block a person from knowing who their own identity is, and has the potential to lead to idol worship of people, addictions and other things.

God tells us in *Isaiah 42:8* That He will not be shared with idols. *I am the Lord: that is my name: and my glory will I not give to another, neither my praise to graven images.*

Armor of God

Agape Love is found in God. It builds us up, helps us blossom, and can help flourish us into stronger, healthier people in mind, body, soul and spirit. An example of Agape Love is Jehovah God and His only begotten son, Jesus Christ who laid down His life for us to have eternal life with Him. Jonathan, King Saul's son, is another example of Agape Love. Jonathan loved David with his whole heart (whole soul) and would lay down his life for David (King David).

1 Samuel 18 1-4. Now when he had finished speaking to Saul, the soul of Jonathan was knit to the soul of David, and Jonathan loved him as his own soul. Saul took him that day, and would not let him go home to his father's house anymore. Then Jonathan and David made a covenant, because he loved him as his own soul. And Jonathan took off the robe that was on him and gave it to David, with his armor, even to his sword and his bow and his belt.

❖ Take a moment in prayer and ask God to break harmful soul-ties of your soul, mind, body and spirit. Write down what you sense the Lord is showing you - whether it was a friend, colleague, family member or something else. Then shout this at the top of your lungs "In the mighty name of Jesus Christ, Soul-Ties and heavy Emotional-ties, get off me and do not return. Lord, forgive me and occupy those places within me so that I can be set-free. Amen!"

The Heart Of God: Fruits Of The Spirit.
Day 11: Love And Joy

The Lord thy God in the midst of thee is mighty; He will save, He will rejoice over thee with joy; He will rest in his love, He will joy over thee with singing.
Zephaniah 3:17

It is no surprise that love, and joy go hand in hand. When you think about a couple who is newly married, joy beams from their faces as they commit to one another in a covenant of love.

That's what God's love does for us. The joy of His Spirit overwhelms us when we enter a covenant relationship with Him. And, when times get tough, we need only to remember that He rejoices over us with joy. He invites us to rest in His love. And He sings over us with exceeding joy.

The fruit of the Spirit is love, joy, peace, patience, kindness, goodness, faithfulness, gentleness and self-control. Against such things there is no law. Galatians 5:22-23 (NKJV)

This means that there is nothing stopping us from thriving in the love and joy of Almighty God - the One who saves, and the One who is Love.

❖ Are you missing joy in your life? Does every day feel like a drudgery? Looking for happiness in counterfeit temporary things can do this. Nothing on this earth can fill the void that only God can do. His can completely fill the void to overflow. This week focus and repeat these words: *The joy of the Lord is my strength* - Psalm 28:7. Write 5 things that brings you true joy.

_____
_____
_____
_____
_____
_____
_____
_____

Day 12: Peace And Reconciliation

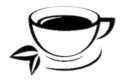

and by Him to reconcile all things to Himself, by Him, whether things on earth or things in heaven, having made peace through the blood of His cross. And you, who once were alienated and enemies in your mind by wicked works, yet now He has reconciled.
Colossians 1:20-21

Oh, the mighty patience of God, that He would bear with us in our sins and pay the penalty for us!

Yet, in our day-to-day interactions, we sometimes forget about His sacrifices. We forget about His forbearance. And, we certainly forget about the peace found only in Him.

Why do we look for satisfaction in other things? We think our "quick fix" will satisfy us, so we constantly look for more. But what we fail to understand is that we CAN have perfect peace ALL the time through Jesus Christ!

Don't you long for that kind of peace in your life more than ever these days?

No longer are we enemies of God by our wicked works. For He has reconciled us unto Himself. He has settled our longing with the most beautiful peace available. And, the best part is, His peace is here to stay.

- ❖ Today, when the storms of life roll in, instead of turning to your ordinary "fix," seek the peace of God. ASK for it! Search the Scriptures for it! Then, rest in the satisfaction of your loving Father. Tell God the type of peace that you seek, and to remove hinderances that block you from it.

_____
_____
_____
_____
_____
_____
_____
_____
_____
_____

Armor of God

Day 13: Kindness And Goodness

If your enemy is hungry, give him bread to eat; And if he is thirsty, give him water to drink; For so you will heap coals of fire on his head, And the Lord will reward you.
Proverbs 25:21-22

We all heard the phrase "kill them with kindness," or "you get more bees with honey!" Although, it is hard to do that when we have been mistreated. However, the Lord guarantees that He will reward us for doing so.

One of the reasons why He warns us about this is because it opens the door to sin and legally allows Satan to harass and torment us. Every chance Satan gets, he aims to cause disruption in our lives because he wants our treasure - our souls! But God tells us how to fight back. *Be ye angry, and sin not: let not the sun go down upon your wrath: Neither give place to the devil. Ephesians 4:26-27*

When we fill our lives with worship, truth, prayer, and things of God, our words and actions will be kind and good. If we are constantly entertaining thoughts that are negative, angry, or self-centered, our words and actions are going to be negative, angry and self-centered.

We need to guard our hearts and minds in Christ Jesus so that we are filled with goodness. Proverbs 4:23-26

- ❖ If you struggle with kindness, and typically allow negative thoughts to circle your mind, change up your routine. Instead of listening to the news in the morning, listen to a Christian podcast. If you usually play secular music in the car, try a worship station instead. Remember, if we consistently put good in, good will come out. Pray for what you feel the Lord is putting on your heart today.

_____
_____
_____
_____
_____
_____

Day 14: Faithfulness

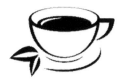

His Lord said unto him, "Well done, good and faithful servant; thou hast been faithful over a few things, I will make thee ruler over many things: enter thou into the joy of thy Lord."
Matthew 25:23

I cannot imagine hearing words more beautiful than, "Well done, good and faithful servant...enter now into the joy of the Lord."

Those are the words every Christian long to hear at the end of their days. Yet, it's one thing to place our faith in Christ for our eternal salvation, but quite another to be faithful in the day-to- day.

Faithfulness is a choice. Every day, when we put our feet to the floor, we CHOOSE whether we will be faithful, even in the small things. Even when things aren't going our way, or we feel stuck in our circumstances, we get to choose to remain faithful.

Armor of God

Yes, the things of this world will pull on our affections, but through the power of the Holy Spirit, we have all the strength in the world to say "NO" to the lusts of the flesh.

Our affections, devotion, and our faithfulness is to Christ alone. For He is worthy of praise.

- ❖ What causes your faith to waiver? Get real with God and real with yourself today. Go to that secret, quiet place and cry out to the Lord. Admit whatever it is that steals your affection and command it to obey your Maker.

_____
_____
_____
_____
_____
_____
_____
_____
_____
_____
_____
_____

Armor of God

Day 15: Gentleness And Self-Control

Let your moderation be known unto all men.
The Lord is at hand.
Philippians 4:5

Self-restraint isn't always easy. People push our buttons. Habits are difficult to break. And sometimes, we just want what we want, not what we feel or believe is the right thing.

But that's the problem with "self" altogether. Trying to break the habit or do the right thing on our own never succeeds for very long. It takes the saturating power of the Holy Spirit and the continuation of His power for us to overcome our habits.

Let your moderation be known to all. Let gentleness and self-control govern your body instead of rash decisions and careless actions. The Lord is at hand. He is not a "far-away" God who is unreachable. In fact, He lives *within* us.

The flesh may seem powerful and too strong to control, but it is, in fact, very weak. It holds no power over us. It has no choice but to surrender to the mighty working of the Holy Spirit's power.

- ❖ Try this exercise today: Ball-up your fists as tight as you can. Hold it tight for ten seconds, then release and watch your hands relax, letting go completely. Turn away from the temptation of the unhealthy habit and towards the Word of God. This is an illustration of submitting your will to the Lord. It shows how you can choose to release your hold and allow the Holy Spirit to produce the fruit of self-control in you.

Spend time in prayer, allowing yourself to let go of the hold. Repeat, "The Holy Spirit is your rear guard."

_____
_____
_____
_____
_____
_____
_____
_____

Armor of God

Renewal
Day 16: Restored And Healed

For I will restore health unto thee, and I will heal thee of thy wounds, saith the Lord; because they called thee an Outcast, saying, This is Zion, whom no man seeketh after.
Jeremiah 30:1

Restoration and renewal comes for every person who puts their hope in the Lord. It does not matter how much of an outcast you have been. It does not matter what people have said about you, believed about you, or done to you. God is your Defender and Healer of your mind, body, soul and spirit!

Psalm 147:2-3 declares that God builds up His people, gathers the outcast, heals the brokenhearted, and binds up their wounds. There is no depth to which we can go where He cannot find us, bring us back to Himself, and restore us. The deeper the sin, the deeper the GRACE!

Do you believe that today?

Know that this physical battle you are in, that there is One who is on the front lines ready to slay the enemy on your behalf. Any wounds you have incurred along the way, He will heal. With the power of His might, and the tender loving grace of His countenance, He will restore health to you.

Declare the Word of God today by remembering these truths:

- ❖ He will restore health unto me.
- ❖ He will heal me of my wounds.

Claim these statements as your own – rewrite them below. Declare them in the face of physical trials. Believe them in the Name of Jesus!

_____
_____
_____
_____
_____
_____

Armor of God

Day 17: The Removal Of Sickness

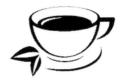

So you shall serve the Lord your God, and He will bless your bread and your water. And I will take sickness away from the midst of you.
Exodus 23:25

Each day we have a decision to make: Who or what are we going to serve?

Will we be self-serving by giving in to every desire? Will we be people-serving by living according to man's expectations? Or, will we serve the Lord?

Devoting our time, energy, and resources to the Living God is the sure path towards balance. Every area of our lives, when committed to the Father, begins to thrive. And there is no stone left unturned when it comes to God's divine blessing.

So, what does it look like to serve God daily?

- ❖ We start the day with Him.

Armor of God

- ❖ We get to know Him through His Word, through prayer, and through worship.
- ❖ We continue the day with Him.

At work, at play, at rest, we structure our lives around the perfect will of the Father. Sometimes, this means denying ourselves or saying "no" to certain things.

- ❖ We end the day with Him.

We go to bed with thankful hearts, resting in His promises and repenting when we sin, knowing He is faithful and just to forgive.

1 John 1:9

Can we trust God to remove sickness from us? We absolutely can. In the trial, discomfort, and illness, continue to serve the Lord in humble faithfulness. Then, watch as His mighty hand of healing works through your body.

- ❖ Write down what times of the day and week do you struggle to be faithful in serving God? Today's challenge is to rearrange your schedule so that those times of struggle will be easy to resist. For example: If evenings are a tempting time to engage in unhealthy activities, start a new activity in the evening that will put a stop to those behaviors. Make the decision to serve God instead of self.

Day 18: The Marvelous Body

"from whom the whole body, joined and knit together by what every joint supplies, according to the effective working by which every part does its share, causes growth of the body for the edifying of itself in love."
Ephesians 4:16

The human body design is so complex. Researchers have said that there are 37.2 trillion cells in the human body – that's more information than can be processed.

But we know that God's infinite wisdom and perfect intelligence is behind every cell ever created. Only He could design such detail in our marvelous bodies. Each part works together because they were joined in perfect harmony. All our organ systems were made to complement each other for optimal wellness.

Just as the body of Christ was designed to work together for growth and edification, so our human bodies were made. And, what we put into these marvelous masterpieces can change all of that. The wrong things we choose to eat, drink, or consume can make us very, very sick. When these things accumulate in the body is when symptoms will manifest. There should be a balance of good foods to keep us healthy, coupled with taking good care of our bodies.

What food choices are you supplying your body with daily? Coffee and donuts? Those will not give your cells the nutrients they need to vitalize your cells.

❖ Take a hard look at the things you KNOW aren't part of God's design for your body. Write it down! Those are the very things that need to go. It's not because you have a Father in heaven who is condemning you. No, you have a loving Father in heaven who wants to make you well! Eradicate the harmful substances that are hindering your growth and destroying your cells.

Armor of God

Day 19: Sustained And Strengthened

The Lord will strengthen him on his bed of illness; You will sustain him on his sickbed.
Psalm 41:3

We live in a time where there are medical treatments for every ailment, and pills for every discomfort and pain – mental and physical. And sometimes, those pills are needed for a time.

However, once we get relief from our symptoms, we tend to forget about our True Healer. It's easy to become dependent on the remedy from our earthly physicians instead of relying on the total healing from the Great Physician.

We are blessed to live in an age of medical breakthroughs. Most of us take for granted the medical provision God has provided. But some of us have become far too dependent on today's health system, forgetting that it is God who sustains us.

God has provided naturally for our physical healing, herbs, vegetables, fruits and water. No one can refute these do not heal the body. All we need to do is take advantage of them and trust the process as our bodies process and distribute the nutrients from these to where they need to go in for our physical healing. The colors, shapes, structures, and aromas of flowers and plants have healing properties that help our souls to heal as well. These are natural workings provided by our incredible God who affords us everything we need to heal.

Any form of sickness should bring us to our knees in surrender. Crying out to God, for the working of His Spirit through our bodies, should be the first form of medication. The Lord will strengthen us in times of illness. He will sustain us and provide the rest and recuperation we need.

❖ Today, plan a half-hour or more to rest. While you are on your bed, thank God for

His healing power. Ask Him to wash over your health and lead you towards what can sustain you. Trust that He will strengthen you. Make this a daily practice of prayer, and rest so you can focus.

Day 20: Every Need

"And my God will meet all your needs according to the riches of his glory in Christ Jesus." Philippians 4:19

Human needs tend to vary from one person to another. Yet, every person has fundamental needs that are hardwired into them from the very moment of conception.

The need for love, assurance, acceptance, and joy, are a few of the fundamental needs of every single person on earth. Sadly, many turn to various vices to fulfill those needs. Things like alcohol, food, drugs, and spending become ways of trying to satisfy our God-given desires.

The sooner we realize that God, the Creator of Heaven and Earth, is the only One who can truly meet our needs, the sooner we will let go of the vices that have strong grips on us. God's riches in Christ Jesus far exceed the temporal satisfactions we feel. Our addictions only satisfy briefly before giving way to feelings of guilt, shame, and defeat.

The cycle can break today by deciding you want to be free, and by declaring that God WILL meet ALL your needs according to the riches of His glory in Christ Jesus.

❖ Write the above passage on 3 separate index cards and post them in prominent places around your space. Every time you are tempted, read the verse aloud. Proclaim it over your life. And most of all, BELIEVE it to be true. God will meet your deepest desires and supply all your needs every single time.

Give praise for the victory!

_____
_____
_____
_____
_____
_____
_____
_____

Armor of God

Mind, Will and Emotions
Day 21: Exhausted Soul

For You formed my inward parts;
You covered me in my mother's womb. I will praise You, for I am fearfully and wonderfully made; Marvelous are Your works,
And that my soul knows very well.
Psalm 139:13-14 (KJV)

Sometimes, it seems that physical healing comes quicker than emotional healing. Perhaps, it's because of the actions we take to assist health, such as taking vitamins, getting fresh air, and drinking plenty of water.

God created three facets in our souls and they are the Mind, Will and Emotions. The Will is where choices, decisions, influence, and the competitive nature are influenced. The Mind is where talents, knowledge, and strategic planning are influenced. The Emotion is where love, compassion and affections are influenced. All three soul facets are connected to the body and spirit and they do affect each other with healing outcomes.

Life's heavy issues or burdens can affect wellness balance in whole or in part, but the grace and mercy of God's Holy Spirit, the Comforter gives rest to the soul by breaking the effects of heaviness. We still will have burdens, but the good news is that they will be light if we ask Jesus. *"Come to Me, all you who labor and are heavy laden, and I will give you rest. Take My yoke upon you and learn from Me, for I am gentle and lowly in heart, and you will find rest for your souls. For My yoke is easy and My burden is light."* Matthew 11:28-30

Are you ready to receive restoration for your soul?

- ❖ What actions can you take to move toward soul wellness? Just like you might take vitamins for physical wellness, inhale the life-giving breath of the Spirit. He longs to lovingly restore you.

Armor of God

Day 22: Soul Care

Beloved, I pray that you may prosper in all things and be in health, just as your soul prospers. 3 John 1:2

What does it mean to nurture our souls? It means to look after, care, and encourage the growth and development of it. Just like a mother, who nurtures her child by providing what he needs, loving him unconditionally, and reaffirming who he was created to be – so, we should care for our own souls. It is a fact that millions of adults were not nurtured when they were children, and that's why as adults, nurture is missing.

The problem is, we don't always know what our souls need. Perhaps, it would be beneficial to start with what they DON'T need:

- ❖ Our souls don't need negative self-talk.
- ❖ Our souls don't need to be ignored.

❖ Our souls don't need to be filled with things that cannot prosper.

When the Bible says that we are to love God with all of our heart, mind, soul, and strength, it reminds us that we are part of a package deal. We are made up of more than just the physical. Therefore, we should pay attention to our whole being and nurture every part.

Careful attention needs to be given to our souls daily. Our souls need nourishment from the truth of God's Word. Positive words of encouragement about who we are in Christ will nurture our soul. We must never separate our physicality with our spirituality. The Lord looks into the depths of our hearts and He wants us to be whole, inside and out.

❖ Do you tend to separate your physical needs and wants with your spiritual ones? Take some time to journal about ways you can nurture your soul. Prayer, worship, reading, and simply resting in God's presence are a few ways to care for and nurture your soul.

Day 23: Isolation

The Lord is near to those who have a broken heart and saves such as have a contrite spirit.
Psalm 34:18

A crucial part of emotional healing is knowing you're not alone. We were created to live in unity with God and harmony with others. Unfortunately, people often isolate themselves when they are hurting. This only leads to more isolation and dependence on substances to fill the void.

The first step in soul-healing is to draw near to God. The Bible says that when we draw near to Him, He draws near to us. (James 4:8) It's important for us to realize that when the Lord seems afar off, it is really us who should spend more time in prayer, bible study and fellowship with Him. Wherever you are, stop and draw near to God. Admit you have wandered away and ask for His loving presence.

The next step in soul-healing is to surround yourself with trustworthy people—preferably believers who will stand with you in the trial and pray for you. Though it may be our tendency to pull away from others, it is absolutely crucial that we resist isolation and find a group of strong friends.

Remember, we were created for community. Communion with God and camaraderie with others is essential to our inner wellbeing.

❖ If you tend to isolate yourself, try today to reach out to 2-3 trusted friends that build you up, and not tare you down. Invited them for a group coffee and discuss your desire to draw closer to them for accountability. Seek strong believers that you sense God is showing you to fellowship with.

_____
_____
_____
_____
_____
_____
_____

Day 24: Walking In God's Presence

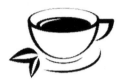

Behold, I will bring it health and healing; I will heal them and reveal to them the abundance of peace and truth.
Jeremiah 33:6

If God can heal and restore a city, a nation, and an entire people group, surely, He can heal our souls. It is His desire to make us whole. He wants nothing more than for us to walk in His presence and live in the light of His truth.

There is an abundance from God that we have yet to tap into. It isn't a secret abundance or a hidden abundance. It is an abundance that was revealed in Jesus Christ. In fact, Jesus Himself said, "I have come that they may have life, and that they may have it more abundantly." (John 10:10)

So, why do we choose to keep living outside of God's abundance?

I believe it is because we have a misconception of the fullness of God. Our flesh is convinced that it needs earthly comforts to be fulfilled, when in reality, those things drain us of abundant life. Peace and truth has been revealed to us. God's lavish banquet of love, peace, joy, and truth are available to us at all times. Yet, so often we search for the crumbs under the table that never satisfy.

He can heal and restore you. Do you believe that today?

❖ What "crumbs" have you settled for in life? What is keeping you from enjoying the abundance of God? Haven't the morsels you've settled for stolen your peace and vitality? Haven't they left you wanting more? Journal about this today and confess whatever is holding you back. Ask for true bread and living water, then He will reveal to you His abundant peace and truth.

_____
_____
_____
_____

Armor of God

Day 25: Hope In God's Promises

And God will wipe away every tear from their eyes; there shall be no more death, nor sorrow, nor crying. There shall be no more pain, for the former things have passed away."
Revelation 21:4

If you were to make a list of your biggest dreams—a bucket list of sorts—what would be the top 3 things you would include? Many of us would write down places we'd like to visit. Perhaps, some of us would record an adventure we'd like to take such as sky-diving or deep-sea diving. Nevertheless, our lists would vary, as each of us has unique ideas of what we'd like to accomplish in our lifetime.

There is one common goal, however, for every believer who has ever lived and will live...the goal of eternal joy with God. We all long for the day when there will be no more death, sorrow, or pain. In fact, we really can't imagine what that will be like.

Surrounded by suffering, it's easy to get downhearted about life. A lot of us feel depressed just by turning on the nightly news. It seems like things are getting worse by the day.

But God!

God, in His infinite wisdom, has promised us a day when He, Himself, will wipe every tear from our eyes. He has given us hope. Our souls can rest in His promises! The big question is, do you know what the promises of God are?

❖ Hold fast to Psalm 9:9-10 when the darkness swirls around you like an ominous cloud. His promises are true and everlasting. On that, our souls can rest. Write down the promises from Psalm 9:9-10, then find 3 more scriptures and write down those promises of God.

_____
_____
_____
_____

Armor of God

Loving Yourself The Way God Loves You
Day 26: Help For Resentment

Love suffers long and is kind; love does not envy; love does not parade itself, is not puffed up; does not behave rudely, does not seek its own, is not provoked, thinks no evil; does not rejoice in iniquity, but rejoices in the truth; bears all things, believes all things, hopes all things, endures all things.
1 Corinthians 13:4-7

Have you ever gone through the stages of forgiveness, only to have something happen and bring back feelings of resentment? Perhaps a reminder of the past resurfaced and all the pain you once suffered was brought to mind. Or, maybe the person who hurt you reentered your life and suddenly you found yourself full of resentment.

What can finally rid a person of past wounds that don't seem to heal?

Armor of God

The answer is simple….*love*.

Love covers over a multitude of things. The Bible says that when we love each other deeply, we actually cover over a multitude of sins. 1 Peter 4:8

The misconception about love is that it is always "warm and fuzzy," never difficult or painful. That simply is not true. Love suffers. Sometimes, it suffers for a long, long time. It isn't easy to love someone who has hurt us. It may even be one of the most difficult things on earth!

But love also heals. Only enduring love closes wounds and eradicates resentment. The question for us is, how will we tap into that enduring love?

❖ From today's Scripture passage, use the list #1 and #2. For list #1, write down all the things that love "does not." For list #2, write down all the things that love "does." Compare the 2 lists and pray for the kind of enduring love that only God can give.

LIST# 1 LOVE DOES NOT	LIST #2 LOVE DOES

Day 27: Overcoming Rejection

For I am persuaded, that neither death, nor life, nor angels, nor principalities, nor powers, nor things present, nor things to come, nor height, nor depth, nor any other creature, shall be able to separate us from the love of God, which is in Christ Jesus our Lord.
Romans 8:38-39

The longing for acceptance, validation, and affirmation lies deep within every human heart. It is a God-given desire, fashioned in us by the Creator who wants an eternal relationship with us.

Unfortunately, we have turned to everything but God for acceptance. And in turn, we have been let down. Man can never fill the void. Eventually, they will fail us, and the wounds of rejection will run deep.

The unconditional love of the Father, displayed in His Son, is our acceptance. Jesus took every rejection to the cross. In the most imaginable love, He willingly bore the hurt and shame for us. And it is through that marvelous love that we are healed from the wounds of rejection.

Will you claim that nothing can separate you from the love of Jesus Christ? Do you believe that?

- ❖ Write a thank you letter to God, specifically thanking Him for his unfailing love. Rejoice in His love of you. Worship Him in Spirit and in truth, knowing that His love is never ending.

_____
_____
_____
_____
_____
_____
_____
_____
_____

Armor of God

Day 28: Overcoming Fear

Fear not: for I have redeemed thee, I have called thee by thy name; thou art mine.
Isaiah 43:1

When we read the words "fear not" in the Bible, we wonder how we are supposed to put them into practice. After all, there are many scary things in this world. Even going to the grocery store puts our lives at risk. We live in a world that is unsafe.

But God!

God, the Father, Son, and Holy Spirit, has redeemed us! He has claimed us as His very own. His loving arm of comfort and protection is consistently around us. We need not fear. Even the mountains could crumble around us and fall into the sea, yet we are upheld by God's righteous right hand.

Armor of God

Fear not, for I am with you; Be not dismayed, for I am your God. I will strengthen you, Yes, I will help you, I will uphold you with My righteous right hand.' Isaiah 41:10

When the Bible says that God, our Redeemer, has called us by name, that indicates a possession. We are God's precious possession! We are His. What a beautiful, comforting thought.

❖ Fear is the absence of faith. Write down what you have been fearing and the things that have caused you torment. Then write down the faith and strength you need in your life to help you overcome fear. Let the Word wash over you with comfort, relieving every bit of fear in your life.

_____
_____
_____
_____
_____
_____
_____
_____
_____

Armor of God

Day 29: Temptation

There hath no temptation taken you but such as is common to man: but God is faithful, who will not suffer you to be tempted above that ye are able; but will with the temptation also make a way to escape, that ye may be able to bear it. 1 Corinthians 10:13

In the Old Testament account of 1 Samuel, chapter 23, David and his men are encircled by King Saul and his men. Fearing for his life, David is hiding in the mountains. When it seems like there is no way out, at the last minute, there is a change in plans. Saul goes to fight another battle. David and his men are spared, and the place is called the Rock of Escape. (see 1 Samuel 23:27-29)

I love that phrase, "Rock of Escape." What a fantastic reminder of who Jesus is for us! In every temptation He makes a way of escape. *Every temptation.*

Armor of God

Only the Rock of your salvation is the way out. There is no unique circumstance where God cannot intervene. Talk to the Lord today about how you feel about your current circumstance, and then watch the Holy Spirit of God lift the effects of it off your soul and spirit. He will show you which way to go. Bless His name!

Prayer Journal:

_____
_____
_____
_____
_____
_____
_____
_____
_____
_____
_____
_____
_____
_____
_____

Armor of God

Day 30: Idolatry

And the residue thereof he maketh a god, even his graven image: he falleth down unto it, and worshippeth it, and prayeth unto it, and saith, Deliver me; for thou art my god.
Isaiah 44:17

Today's devotion is a serious one. In fact, I ask you to read Isaiah 44:17 again. It portrays a person fashioning an idol, carving details into it and then falling down to worship. We might think this verse has nothing to do with us. After all, we don't carve images to bow down to.

But think about this: Some of us stock our refrigerators with things we crave and cannot do without. We bow down to them and worship them in the sense that we think about them, plan for them, and indulge freely in them. For others, it's the medicine cabinet full of "go-to" fixes. A pill for this, a pill for that, and all our troubles are washed down with a glass of water. Yet, for others, their idols are people. They exalt certain people in their lives, even those who are bad for them. Their devotion is to a person rather than to God.

Each one of us struggles with the tendency towards idolatry. Anything can be "carved" into an image to worship. But our idols cannot and will not deliver us. No matter how much affection and attention we give them, they have no power.

Turn to the Mighty Deliverer of your heart, mind, soul and strength! Repent of the idols you have stashed away—the idols that have a hold of your affections. Our merciful God is faithful and just to forgive. (1 John 1:9)

- ❖ Get away from your idols today by taking a walk or even a drive. Pray for God to reveal any and every person or thing that has caused you to bow down in idolatry. Ask for the cleansing power of the Holy Spirit. Then, when you return home, make the decision to throw the idols away. If it's a toxic person that has become an idol in your life, decide to end the relationship.

Armor of God

Abiding In Christ
Day 31: Condemnation Or Conviction?

There is therefore now no condemnation
to them which are in Christ Jesus,
who walk not after the flesh,
but after the Spirit.
Romans 8:1

Feelings of condemnation can mask the truth of what Christ has done in the life of a believer. Unworthiness, shame, and guilt can overshadow God's grace, love, and forgiveness. There is a difference between condemnation and conviction. God's Spirit convicts us of wrong-doing so that we will turn from it and walk in His ways. Condemnation is from the enemy, saying, "You are worthless. You might as well give up."

Choosing to walk in-step with the Holy Spirit is a deliberate, daily decision. The flesh will pull on our affections every time. And when we give in to the flesh, feelings of condemnation will sweep in, not from the Holy Spirit, but from Satan.

Let's break free from every form of condemnation by shaking off everything that is opposed to God. Let's walk in accordance with the Holy Spirit, chasing after things that are good, righteous and holy.

❖ Write the word "CONDEMNATION" in big letters. Then, list several words that describe condemnation. Now, list several words that describe the opposite of condemnation. Do you see the difference how much God loves you? Use this as a reminder how much Jesus Christ loves you when the enemy tries to attack you with condemnation.

_____
_____
_____
_____
_____
_____
_____
_____

Armor of God

Day 32: What Your Heart Desires

If you abide in Me, and My words abide in
you, you will ask what you desire,
and it shall be done for you.
John 15:7

To "abide" means to *remain, reside,* and *stay.* It is an action word that indicates movement in a person's life. This may seem contrary to the thought of remaining still, but it's an action on our part nonetheless. Think of it this way: If we decide to remain in our seat even though we would rather get up and leave, we are acting upon the decision to stay. We are making a move to *remain* in our seat. So, it is with Jesus. We remain in Him even when people try to change our focus. We remain even when things get difficult.

Abiding in Christ means that we abide in His words. We allow His words to do a mighty work in us, changing us from the inside out. We adopt His precepts as our own. We declare His truth and hold fast to it. And by His words, we are transformed.

Abiding means we begin to desire what He desires. We crave the True Bread He offers. We thirst for Living Water. And, we begin to ask for things according to His will and not our own. The is how the verse in John 15 comes to pass. We ask what we desire, and He gives it, not because He fulfills all of our wishes, but because our desires align fully with His.

- ❖ Do you sometimes view God as a "genie in a bottle"? Perhaps, you are in the habit of asking Him for things that are not in accordance with His will. Then, when He doesn't answer, you feel rejected. Today, ask God for things that align with His will and His Word. Then you can be assured He will give you your heart's desires.

Day 33: Faithful

But you are not in the flesh but in the Spirit, if indeed the Spirit of God dwells in you. Now if anyone does not have the Spirit of Christ, he is not His. And if Christ is in you, the body is dead because of sin, but the Spirit is life because of righteousness.
Romans 8:9-10

Faith is spiritual, it is not physical. It comes by hearing the word of God. *So then faith cometh by hearing, and hearing by the word of God. Romans 10:17.*

There is a misconception in the believer's life that Jesus comes and goes, sometimes filling us with His Spirit and sometimes leaving us on our own. This simply is not true. Remember, God is faithful no matter what. We are the ones who pull away, ignore Him, and take our own paths.

The Bible says, *"If we are faithless, He remains faithful; for He cannot deny Himself."* 2 Timothy 2:13

Does this mean that it is OK for us to be faithless or to live how we want, knowing He will remain faithful? Not at all! For it is by faith that we are able to live and abide in Christ, our Rock and Redeemer.

Are you ready to strap faith to your spirit by reading the word of God and actively living every day in its strength and wisdom? Aren't you ready to live fully alive because Christ is in you. Cling wholeheartedly to Him and you will be lifted above the addiction and it will no longer have its grip on you.

- ❖ Take a minute in prayer and shout your victory today. Call upon the One who resides in you from the moment you first saw the light. Know that He is there, guiding your life in righteousness. Remember that He lives in you and remains faithful.

_____
_____
_____

Armor of God

Day 34: Born Again

Jesus answered, "Most assuredly, I say to you, unless one is born of water and the Spirit, he cannot enter the kingdom of God. That which is born of the flesh is flesh, and that which is born of the Spirit is spirit. Do not marvel that I said to you, 'You must be born again.'
John 3:5-7

A Jewish ruler and scholar came to Jesus at night to inquire of Him. And when the Lord told him how he could enter the kingdom of God, the ruler could not grasp the meaning. *"How can a man be born when he is old? Can he enter a second time into his mother's womb and be born?" John 3:4.*

Be born again is crucial for our daily walk with God. The flesh only produces dead works, but the Spirit produces life and is a direct channel of communication between God and us.

When our first parents, Adam and Eve sinned against God in the Garden of Eden, they acted out of their flesh and not from faith. They ate the fruit from the Tree of Knowledge of Good and Evil that God told them not to - *Genesis Chapter 2 and 3.*

That sin prompted God to remove Adam and Eve from the Garden of Eden so that they would not eat from the Tree of Life in this garden. That would have made it possible for Adam and Eve, including all of mankind to live FOREVER in sin on this earth. Satan himself wanted this because he wanted mankind to exalt him above God our creator.

Adam and Eve's sin caused their covenant relationship with God to be removed, but for us, the only thing that could restore us back to it was God's only begotten Son, Jesus Christ. That is why we must be born of the Spirit because the flesh is corrupted with sin.

Thank God for Jesus taking our sins on Himself at Calvary so that we can have covenant relationship and everlasting life with the Father.

Do not be confused by the flesh. Simply realize that the flesh pulls in every kind of direction—discouragements, strongholds, habits and addictions—but there is life in the Holy Spirit of God who overcomes all the devices of the flesh (Satan's playground).

- ❖ If you aren't sure if you've been born again, don't wait another day to meet with a trusted pastor. Be honest. Ask questions. And most of all, pray for re-birth by the glorious Spirit of God, that you might be truly born again.

Prayer to be born again:

_____
_____
_____
_____
_____
_____
_____
_____
_____
_____

Armor of God

Day 35: True Identity

And God said, "Let us make man in our image, after our likeness: and let them have dominion over the fish of the sea, and over the fowl of the air, and over the cattle, and over all the earth, and over every creeping thing that creepeth upon the earth."
Genesis 1:26

There seems to be a desperate search, nowadays, for people to find their true identity. But the answer has always resided in our covenant relationship with God. In **Him** is where we fit, belong, and see clearly our purpose in life.

The covenant relationship that Adam and Eve had with God was a sweet fellowship of true friendship and family. They shared a bond like no other. Adam and Eve knew who they were, and whose they were. See Genesis 1:26-31, 2:1-25.

Armor of God

1. Adam's assignment and position were to have dominion over all the earth and take care of it. Genesis 1:26.
2. Adam's identity was found ONLY in his association, the covenant relationship with God.
3. Adam's purpose on earth was to be fruitful a multiply.
4. Adam's position was the assignment given by God.
5. His significance was that he was important, and a friend of God.

These truths are foundational to our existence! We so easily forget that we are made in the very image of the Lord! We are *like* Him. Our whole identity and purpose are found in Him. When we grasp that, even a little, our whole perspective on life begins to change.

❖ Write down what or whom have you placed your identity in? Is it in your wealth or status? Is it in your abilities or strengths? Commit, today, to finding your TRUE identity in the Lord Jesus Christ. For it is in Him that you live and move and have your being. Acts 17:28

Motivational Gifts. Finding Your Calling
Day 36: Makeover

Therefore if any man be in Christ, he is a new creature: old things are passed away; behold, all things are become new.
2 Corinthians 5:17

Have you ever seen one of those "makeover" shows, where they take the frumpy, middle-aged woman, who has gotten into a fashion rut, and turned her into a glamorous looking lady?

Many of us dream of having a new start or a complete makeover. We long to stop living in the cycle of good days/bad days. Some of us might even dream of running away to start fresh!

But in Christ, we are made **brand new every single day**. Better than any makeover, we are transformed inside and out. Each morning, we have the opportunity to say, *"Here I am, Lord, now do Your mighty work in me."*

Will you say that today?

There are old things in your life that need to go. There are closets that need to be cleaned out and things thrown away. I'm not talking about our physical closets full of clothes, shoes, and such. I'm talking about our spiritual closets of hidden things that don't belong.

"Behold! All things have become new!" Aren't you longing to proclaim that today?

- ❖ Write that phrase. Declare that all things have become new in Christ Jesus. Rid your life of all old things that absolutely MUST go. You can do it! Write down what you sense the Lord is telling you to release.

_____
_____
_____
_____
_____
_____
_____

Day 37: Are You A Proclaimer?

There was a man sent from God, whose name was John. The same came for a witness, to bear witness of the Light, that all men through him might believe. He was not that Light, but was sent to bear witness of that Light.
John 1:6-8

Are you a Proclaimer? Are you a natural at declaring, announcing, and demonstrating what you believe in?

Perhaps, you have the same motivational gift of John the Baptist. From birth, he was set apart to prepare the way for the Lord. Can you imagine such a calling? Even living in the desert and surviving on locusts and wild honey, you could say that John was "all in!"

Filled with the Holy Spirit in his mother's womb (Luke 1:15). His mission was to prepare the hearts of people to receive the Messiah. His message was one of repentance and restoration. He wasn't afraid of the Pharisees and what they might do to stop him. He was faithful and mighty for God—a proclaimer of truth to all who would hear.

Does John's example resonate with you? What things would you love to proclaim for the sake of Christ? What is stopping you from sharing that message with the world?

This is the day to rise up, out of your comfort zone, and proclaim the day of salvation. And the Bible says, THIS is the day of salvation!

"In an acceptable time I have heard you, And in the day of salvation I have helped you." Behold, now is the accepted time; behold, now is the day of salvation. 2 Corinthians 6:2.

❖ If you know, in the depths of your soul, that you are a "Proclaimer for God," rise up to the challenge today. Make a list of things you KNOW you need to tell the world. Then, take one actionable step in doing that today.

Day 38: Are You A Server?

Now it came to pass, as they went, that
he entered into a certain village: and
a certain woman named Martha
received him into her house.
Luke 10:38

If you have a servant's heart, you've experienced the joy of inviting people into your home and making them feel comfortable. It comes natural to you to offer a cup of coffee or glass of iced-tea and make people feel right at home.

Please don't underestimate this motivational gift! It is a beautiful gift from the Holy Spirit and much needed in our world today. Unfortunately, hospitality has faded away in our society, as people have become too busy to interact with one another. Serving people has sadly been forsaken in favor of self-service.

The best part about the gift of server, is that it gets the focus off of ourselves and off of our strongholds. It turns our attention to the needs of others and therefore brings balance to our lives. Here are a couple of ideas for serving others:

- ❖ Consider hosting this bible study at church. It would be a learning experience for everyone!
- ❖ Host a greet and meet your neighbors at a neighborhood coffee shop to get to your neighbors. You never know what relationships are waiting to be cultivated right around the corner!
- ❖ Write down more ideas that interest you and could bring balance to your life.

_____
_____
_____
_____
_____
_____
_____
_____
_____
_____
_____

Armor of God

Day 39: Are You A Teacher?

Give instruction to a wise man, and he will be yet wiser: teach a just man, and he will increase in learning.
Proverbs 9:9

This gift is Teacher of Teachers. The heart of a teacher is often generous, selfless, and nurturing. The desire to pass on knowledge and offer instruction resides deep within the gifted teacher's soul. Praise the Lord for such a valuable gift for the body of Christ!

In 2 Timothy 1:11, Paul shares that he was "appointed as a herald, an apostle, and a teacher." He was appointed by God to share the Good News of Jesus Christ, lead other Christians, and teach people about the ways of God.

Wow! What a divine calling!

You are called according to the divine purpose of God. And when He called you to teach, He gives you wisdom, knowledge, and insight to do it. You need not hold back or be intimidated by your own insecurities. You need simply to get into the Word of God and learn everything you can so that you can go out and share it with the world!

- ❖ What do you think? Is this your motivational gift? Perhaps, you are appointed, just like Paul, to teach people about Christ. Today, spend some time writing down the Good News of the Gospel. Imagine there is a loved one sitting across from you who desperately needs to hear the truth. How would you teach it to them?

_____
_____
_____
_____
_____
_____
_____
_____
_____
_____
_____
_____

Armor of God

Day 40: Are You An Exhorter?

Till I come, give attendance to reading,
to exhortation, to doctrine. Neglect
not the gift that is in thee...
1 Timothy 4:13-14

An exhorter walks alongside others and gives encouragement, advice, or counsel. To be filled with the gift of exhortation means that building others up comes naturally to you. It is *in* you to encourage others who are down-and-out. It is part of who you are to give wise counsel.

Barnabas was named, in the book of Acts, as the "son of encouragement." Perhaps a prophetic name, Barnabas was an active part of edifying some of the first believers in Christ.

Then tidings of these things came unto the ears of the church which was in Jerusalem: and they sent forth Barnabas, that he should go as far as Antioch. Who, when he came, and had seen the grace of God, was glad, and exhorted them all, that with purpose of heart they would cleave unto the Lord. For he was a good man, and full of the Holy Ghost and of faith: and much people was added unto the Lord. Acts 11:22-24

What a beautiful description of a life lived within his motivational gift!

Is exhortation something the Lord has pressed upon your heart? Are you actively pursuing it? Here are a few ideas to hopefully inspire you to put your Spiritual gift of exhortation into practice:

- ❖ Call or email someone who has been on your heart recently. Remind them of the goodness of God and encourage them in the faith.
- ❖ Send a handwritten card or letter to a loved one. Encourage them by pointing out several things you love about them.
- ❖ Consider starting or joining an "Exhortation Team" in your church. Meet weekly to discuss ways in which you can encourage other believers.

_____

_____

Armor of God

Day 41: Are You A Giver?

"If you take the left, then I will go to
the right; or, if you go to the
right, then I will go to the left."
Genesis 13:9

Abraham was a giver. More concerned about relationships than acquiring land or wealth, he gave from a spirit of generosity. At one point, when it came time for Abraham and his nephew, Lot, to go their separate ways, Abraham gave Lot first choice of the land. Lot, seeing that the plains of the Jordan were well-watered like a beautiful garden, chose to settle there. And, without question, Abraham accepted it.

Are you a giver? Has God instilled in you a motivational gift to be generous with your time, talent, and treasure?

What an opportunity of divine blessing you have for others! Don't let the enemy stand in the way of sharing your wisdom and resources with those in need. Here are a few ways to inspire your motivational gift of giving.

- ❖ Join a "race for the cause" and reap some physical benefits while giving to a worthy cause in your community.
- ❖ Help a single mom in your church or neighborhood. Even babysitting for an evening can be a huge way to give.
- ❖ Offer to mentor a younger woman in the faith. Meet for coffee and study the Bible together.
- ❖ Cook a meal for a family in need.
- ❖ Write down what you sense the Lord will have you do for others.

_____
_____
_____
_____
_____
_____
_____
_____
_____
_____
_____
_____

Armor of God

Day 42: Are You An Administrator?

For the administration of this service not only supplieth the want of the saints, but is abundant also by many thanksgivings unto God...
2 Corinthians 9:12

Imagine what our world would be like without administrators to organize and delegate? I'm afraid chaos would ensue, and we would be left with an ineffective mess in the home and the workplace.

So, it is in the Christian life as well. The motivational gift of administration, which was displayed in Joseph's life, is a gift that the body of Christ cannot do without. Here's an example of Joseph's gift in action:

So the advice was good in the eyes of Pharaoh and in the eyes of all his servants. And Pharaoh said to his servants, "Can we find such a one as this, a man in whom is the Spirit of God? Then Pharaoh said to Joseph,

"Inasmuch as God has shown you all this, there is no one as discerning and wise as you. You shall be over my house, and all my people shall be ruled according to your word; only in regard to the throne will I be greater than you." And Pharaoh said to Joseph, "See, I have set you over all the land of Egypt." Genesis 41:27-41

The most miraculous part about Joseph's rise to power wasn't because he was a gifted administrator, but because he was faithful to God in the midst of the worst of circumstances. Joseph had been in prison and seemingly long-forgotten. But, when the time was right, and his gifts were needed, he was faithful to walk in them. In turn, Joseph was highly favored of God and by the ruler of Egypt.

- ❖ Be prepared to move forward in your administrative gifts and watch the Lord do a mighty work in you!
- ❖ Write down what you sense the Lord is leading you to do in your life.

_____
_____
_____
_____

Armor of God

Day 43: Are You Compassionate?

Therefore, as the elect of God, holy and beloved, put on tender mercies, kindness, humility, meekness, longsuffering;
Colossians 3:12

It cannot be stressed enough, the importance of compassion in today's culture. With the explosion of the internet, and people's ability to write whatever they want across the World Wide Web, the need for compassion is greater than ever.

Has God gifted you with a heart of compassion? Do you relate to the Good Samaritan, in the Bible, who was the only one to stop and help someone in need? Take a look.

Then Jesus answered and said: "A certain man went down from Jerusalem to Jericho, and fell among thieves, who stripped him of his clothing, wounded him, and departed, leaving him half dead. Now by chance a certain priest came down that road. And when he saw him, he passed by on the other side. Likewise a Levite, when he arrived at the place, came and looked, and passed by on the other side. But a certain Samaritan, as he journeyed, came where he was. And when he saw him, he had compassion. Luke 10:30-33.

The least likely person was the one to stop and help. Compassion resided in him and he couldn't help but offer assistance. Does compassion reside in you? Are you especially sensitive to the needs of others?

Fan that gift into flame and let compassion take over as you allow God to work through you. It may be your God-given ministry and bring balance to your life! Walk in your motivational gift and know that you are meeting needs that no one else will.

- ❖ Consider starting a "Compassionate Care" ministry at your church and gather together likeminded believers to join you in showing compassion to others.
- ❖ Write the steps you can take to do it and pray about it

Armor of God

Day 44: Are You A Helper?

And God has appointed these in the church: first apostles, second prophets, third teachers, after that miracles, then gifts of healings, helps, administrations, varieties of tongues.
1 Corinthians 12:28

The motivational gift of "helps" is often overshadowed by others in the church body that are more prominent and in the forefront. But really, it's those behind-the-scenes acts of service that hold the body together and keep its wheels turning.

Community work days, church clean-up days, and even painting days at the local elementary school are things that gifted helpers are most good at. Do you get excited just thinking about putting your strengths into action? Perhaps, you are a helper like Tabitha, in the Bible, who was full of good works unto the Lord.

Now there was at Joppa a certain disciple named Tabitha, which by interpretation is called Dorcas: this woman was full of good works and almsdeeds (charitable deeds) which she did. Acts 9:36

If being a helper is your motivational gift, do not despise it. Be encouraged today and rise up with assurance that your gift is mightily needed. Helps is what gives structure and stability to all the other gifts. And it is a gift to be thankful for. Here are some things you can consider.

- ❖ Volunteering for a "helps" related event. Use your strengths for the glory of God. It won't take you long to find someone in need of exactly what you can give.
- ❖ Help your church distribute food and supplies to the community.
- ❖ Become a greeter at church.
- ❖ List some other things you sense the Lord is leading you to do and pray about it.

_____
_____
_____
_____
_____
_____
_____

Day 45: Are You An Intercessor?

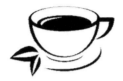

For I know that this shall turn to my salvation through your prayer, and the supply of the Spirit of Jesus Christ.
Philippians 1:19

Although prayer is part of every Christian's life, it is also a mighty gift when used to intercede on behalf of others. There are certain people who the Lord has blessed with the heart and motivation for intercessory prayer. They are the people who go to their knees often, in that secret quiet place, and pour out their petitions to God.

Are you an intercessor? When you say that you will pray for someone, do you drop everything to do it? Are you called to say a prayer for random people you see on the street? Do you spend ample time in your prayer closet?

This gift is precious! Without intercession, Christians would be living very discouraged lives. For our prayers rise as incense before the

Armor of God

throne of God and He hears us when we cry out to Him.

Let my prayer be set forth before thee as incense; and the lifting up of my hands as the evening sacrifice. Psalm 141:2

Think about how blessed you feel when someone has prayed for you. It means so much to us when we know others are taking the time to speak to the Lord on our behalf, doesn't it? Let's value the intercessor greatly, knowing that they are invaluable to the body of Christ.

If you are an intercessor, please do not dismiss the importance of your gift. Continue in it, steadfast, without wavering. People need your prayers!

❖ Spend time in prayer, thanking God for this incredible gift. Ask Him to help you walk in in and lead you.

_____
_____
_____
_____
_____

Armor of God

RESOURCES AND REFERENCES

80 Toxic Food Ingredients

The following ingredients used in excess have been historically known to contribute to organ stress. See the Environmental Working Group at Ewg.Org for the kinds of stress.

1. Acesulfame-K (Acesulfame Potassium)
2. Acetylated Esters Of Mono- And Diglycerides
3. Ammonium Chloride
4. Artificial Colors
5. Artificial Flavors
6. Artificial Preservatives
7. Aspartame
8. Azodicarbonamide
9. Benzoate
10. Benzoyl Peroxide
11. BHA (Butylated Hydroxyanisole)
12. BHT (Butylated Hydroxytoluene)
13. Bleached Flour
14. Bromated Flour
15. Brominated Vegetable Oil (BVO)
16. Calcium Bromate
17. Calcium Disodium EDTA
18. Calcium Peroxide

19. Calcium Propionate
20. Calcium Saccharin
21. Calcium Sorbate
22. Calcium Stearoyl-2-Lactylate
23. Caprocaprylobehenin
24. Carmine
25. Certified Colors
26. Cyclamates
27. Dimethylpolysiloxane
28. Dioctyl Sodium Sulfosuccinate (DSS)
29. Disodium Calcium EDTA
30. Disodium Dihydrogen EDTA
31. Disodium Guanylate
32. Disodium Inosinate
33. EDTA
34. Ethoxyquin
35. Ethyl Vanillin
36. Ethylene Oxide
37. FD & C Colors
38. FD&C Blue, Green, Red, Yellow Dyes and Lakes (all Numbers#)
39. Foie Gras
40. GMP (Disodium Guanylate)
41. High Fructose Corn Syrup
42. Hydrogenated Fats (oils)
43. IMP (Disodium Inosinate)
44. Irradiated Foods
45. Lactylated Esters Of Mono- And Diglycerides

46. Lead Soldered Cans
47. Methyl Silicon
48. Methylparaben
49. Microparticularized Whey Protein Derived Fat Substitute
50. Monosodium Glutamate (MSG)
51. Natamycin
52. Nitrates/Nitrites
53. Partially Hydrogenated Oil
54. Polydextrose
55. Potassium Benzoate
56. Potassium Bisulfite
57. Potassium Bromate
58. Potassium Metabisulfite
59. Potassium Sorbate
60. Propionates
61. Propyl Gallate
62. Propylparaben
63. Saccharin
64. Sodium Aluminum Sulfate
65. Sodium Benzoate
66. Sodium Bisulfite
67. Sodium Diacetate
68. Sodium Glutamate
69. Sodium Nitrate/Nitrite
70. Sodium Propionate
71. Sodium Stearoyl-2-Lactylate
72. Sodium Sulfite
73. Sorbic Acid

74. Sucralose
75. Sucroglycerides
76. Sucrose Polyester
77. Sulfites (Sulfur Dioxide)
78. TBHQ (Tertiary Butylhydroquinone)
79. Tetrasodium EDTA
80. Vanillin

U.S.A. Christian Drug Recovery Centers

Alabama
(call the centers to confirm)

Name Of Christian Rehab	Gender	Program Length	Contact	Website Address
Life Challenge / Teen Challenge	Adults And Teen	1 Year	417-581-2181	Teenchal-lengeusa.Com
Canaan Land Ministries	Men	1 Year	334-365-2200	Canaanland.Com
Restoration Ranch	Adults	Long-Term	256-381-0930	Missionteens.Com
Wellspring	Women		(334)365-9086	
Rapha Ministries	Men	6 Month To 1year	256-538-7458	Raphaministries.Net
The Lovelady Center	Women /Children		205-833-7410	Loveladycenter.Org
Faith Rescue Mission			334-262-6024	Faithrescue.Org

Armor of God

Salvation Army (Arc)	Adults	6 To 9 Mo.	800-728-7825	Satruck.Org
The Foundry Men's / Women's Recovery	Adults	12-18 Months	205-424-Hope X4673	Thefoundryonline.Org

Arkansas
(call the centers to confirm)

Name Of Christian Rehab	Gender	Program Length	Contact	Website Address
Life Challenge / Teen Challenge	Adults And Teen	1 Year	417-581-2181	Teenchallengeusa.Com
John 3:16 Ministry	Men	Long-Term	870-799-2525	John316ministry.Com
God's New Life Mbtc	Adults	Long-Term	870-358-4851	Missionteens.Com
Grace Mbtc	Adults	Long-Term	870-573-6414	Missionteens.Com
Capstone	Youth		866-729-4479 501-729-4479	Capstonetreatmentcenter.Com
Salvation Army (Arc)	Adults	6 To 9 Mo.	800-728-7825	Satruck.Org

California

Name Of Christian Rehab	Gender	Program Length	Contact	Website Address
Life Challenge/ Teen	Adults And Teen Programs	1 Year	417-581-2181	Teenchallengeusa.Com

Challenge				
Dream Center	Adults	1 Year	213-273-7000	Dreamcenter.Org
New Life Spirit Recovery	Adults	Short-Term	714-841-1906	Newlifespiritrecovery.Com
Salvation Army (Arc)	Adults	6 To 9 Mo.	800-728-7825	Satruck.Org
Dream Center Teen Discipleship	Teens	Long-Term	213-273-7210	
Mountain Of Mercy Mbtc	Adults	Long-Term	707-601-3403	Missionteens.Com
House Of Miracles			951-334-9991	
Advent Group Ministries	Teens		408-281-0708	Adventgm.Org
His Way Recovery House	Adults		209-401-9126	Hiswayrecovery.Org
U Turn For Christ Camino	Men	2 Months +	530-644-1982	Uturnforchrist-camino.Com
U Turn For Christ	Men/Women	2 Months +	951-943-7097 Or 951-928-3002	Uturnforchrist.Com
U Turn For Christ Needles		2 Months +	760-326-5999	Uturnforchrist.Com
U Turn For Christ Trinidad		2 Months +	868-667-8345	
New Life For Girls	Women	Long-Term	559-486-2515	Newlifeforgirls.Org
Set Free	Men & Women		Men: 951-849-3678 Women: 951-849-1211	Setfreerocks.Com
Calvary Ranch	Men	Short Term	800-404-2258	Calvaryranch.Org

Armor of God

Victory Outreach (Many Locations)	Adults	1 Year	(909) 599-4437	Victoryoutreach.Org
Christian Life Discipleship Program	Men/Women	6 Months	213-347-6300	Urm.Org
Walter Hoving Home	Women	6 Months To 1 Year	626-405-0950	
Lighthouse Recovery Program	Women & Child		805-385-7200	Vcrescuemission.Org
Ventura County Rescue Mission Recovery Program	Men		805-436-4591	Vcrescuemission.Org
Mercy Ministries	Women	Long Term	615-831-6987	Mercyministries.Org
True Vines Men's Home	Men		909-884-7087	

Colorado
(call the centers to confirm)

Name Of Christian Rehab	Gender	Program Length	Contact	Website Address
Life Challenge/ Teen Challenge	Adults And Teen Programs	1 Year	417-581-2181	Teenchallengeusa.Com
U Turn For Christ	Men	2 Months +	(719) 473-6285	Uturnforchrist.Com
Salvation Army (Arc)	Adults	6 To 9 Mo.	800-728-7825	Satruck.Org
Victory Outreach	Adults	1 Year	719 477-0000 719-584-7722 303-455-7410 303-937-	Victoryoutreach.Org

Devina H. Collier, Biblical Naturopath

			7460 970-351-6544	
Christian Discipleship Center	For Native American Christians	90-Day	970-565-3290	C-D-C.Org

Connecticut
(call the centers to confirm)

Name Of Christian Rehab	Gender	Program Length	Contact	Website Address
Life Challenge/ Teen Challenge	Adults And Teen Programs	1 Year	417-581-2181	Teenchallengeusa.Com
Salvation Army (Arc)	Adults	6 To 9 Mo.	800-728-7825	Satruck.Org

Delaware

Name Of Christian Rehab	Gender	Program Length	Contact	Website Address
Life Challenge/ Teen Challenge	Adults And Teen Programs	1 Year	417-581-2181	Teenchal-lengeusa.Com
Salvation Army (Arc)	Adults	6 To 9 Mo.	800-728-7825	Satruck.Org

Florida

Name Of Christian Rehab	Gender	Program Length	Contact	Website Address

Name	Population	Duration	Phone	Website
Jacksonville Teen Challenge	Adult Men	1 Year	904-398-0013	Jacksonville.Teen-challenge.Cc
Teen Challenge	Adults	1 Year	417-862-6969	Teenchallengeusa.Com
Center Of Hope	Adults	6 Months To 1 Year	727-729-8399	Centerofhopedtc.Org
Jesus Is	Adults	90 Days	352-447-2731	Jesusis.Com
Sonrise	Adults	Long-Term	954-485-0951	Missionteens.Com
Agape Home	Women & Children		863-946-2228	Agapehome.Org
Calvary House	Men	Long-Term	954-943-8328	Calvaryhouseftl.Com
Lifebuilders Recovery Program In Jax	Men/Women	Long-Term	904-421-5169	Crmjax.Org
New Life Dream Center	Men	Long-Term	239.274.8881 Ext 231	Newlifedreamcenters.Com
New Life Dream Center	Women	Long-Term	239.274.8881 Ext 243	Newlifedreamcenters.Com
Harvest Vineyard Ministries	Men/Women	1 Year	850-682-6447	Harvestvineyard.Org
Faith Farm	Women	9 Months	561-732-2370	Faithfarm.Org
Faith Farm	Men	9 Months	561-733-7262 954-463-6214	Faithfarm.Org

			863-763-4224	
Liberty Lodge	Men	8 Months +	(321) 264-0757 (321) 267-3646	Libertylodgeministries.Com
Hosanna Ministries	Men		321-804-4919	Thechristinyou.Net
His Place Ministries	Men	Long-Term	321-674-9009	
Dunklin Memorial Camp	Men	9 Months	772-597-2841	Dunklin.Org
Open Homes Regeneration	Men	9 Months	407-382-7962	Openhomesregeneration.Com
Salvation Army (Arc)	Adults	6 To 9 Mo.	800-728-7825	Satruck.Org
Christian Care Center	Men	1 Year	352-787-9904	Christiancarecenter.Org
Women's Care Center	Women	1 Year	352-787-8929	Christiancarecenter.Org
Victory Outreach	Adults	1 Year	407 521-2195 813-932-3821 (305-636-5311 Hispanic)	Victoryoutreach.Org
Youth Challenge	Youth		352-748-5595	Ycofflorida.Com
Fresh Start Ministries	Men	1 Year	407-293-3822	

Armor of God

Name	Gender	Program Length	Contact	Website Address
Women's Refuge: After Rehab	Women		904-810-4911 772-770-4424	Womensrefugevb.Org
Lifeline	Men/Women	90 Days	904-355-1205	Trinityrescue.Org
The Refuge Ranch	Women	Long-Term	772-597-0992	Therefugeranch.Org

Georgia
(call the centers to confirm)

Name Of Christian Rehab	Gender	Program Length	Contact	Website Address
Life Challenge/ Teen Challenge	Adults And Teen Programs	1 Year	417-581-2181	Teenchallengeusa.Com
The Apostles House	Men	6 Month To Year	478-864-7558	Apostleshouse.X10host.Com
Angles In Flight	Women	6 Month To Year	478-864-8090	Angelsinflight13.Org
Salvation Army (Arc)	Adults	6 To 9 Mo.	800-728-7825	Satruck.Org
Victory Outreach	Adults	1 Year	404-762-1602	Victoryoutreach.Org
My Sister's House	Women	Long-Term	404-367-2465	Atlantamission.Org
The Potter's House	Men	Long-Term	706-543-8338 X5103	Atlantamission.Org
Mbtc	Adults	Long-Term	912-234-7000	Missionteens.Com
Victory Home	Men	25 Weeks	706-754-6030	Victoryhome.Org
The	Men		912-529-6712	Cfcnewlife.Org

Christian Family Center				
Providence Ministries	Men & Women	6 Month	706-275-0268	Providenceministriesinc.Com
New Beginnings In Christ	Men		478-763-2647	Nbicrecovery.Com
The Anchorage	Men		229-435-5692	Anchorageofalbany.Org
No Longer Bound	Men	1 Year	770-886-7873	Nolongerbound.Com
Penfield Christian Homes	Men	Six Weeks	866-542-5378	Penfieldrecovery.Com

Hawaii
(call the centers to confirm)

Name Of Christian Rehab	Gender	Program Length	Contact	Website Address
Life Challenge / Teen Challenge	Adults And Teen Programs	1 Year	417-581-2181	Teenchallengeusa.Com
U-Turn For Christ	Adults		951-204-2165	Uturnforchristkauai.Com
Salvation Army (Arc)	Adults	6 To 9 Mo.	800-728-7825	Satruck.Org
Victory Outreach	Adults	1 Year	808 681-0381	Victoryoutreach.Org
Salvation Army Addiction Trt / Detox Services	Adults		(808) 595-6371	Salvationarmyhawaii.Com

Idaho
(call the centers to confirm)

Name Of Christian Rehab	Gender	Program Length	Contact	Website Address
Life Challenge / Teen Challenge	Adults And Teen Programs	1 Year	417-581-2181	Teenchallengeusa.Com
Salvation Army (Arc)	Adults	6 To 9 Mo.	800-728-7825	Satruck.Org

Illinois

Name Of Christian Rehab	Gender	Program Length	Contact	Website Address
Life Challenge / Teen Challenge	Adults And Teen Programs	1 Year	417-581-2181	Teenchallengeusa.Com
Reformers Unanimous Residential	Adults	6 Months	866-733-6768	Ruhomes.Org
First Fruits	Adults	Long-Term	618-498-3560	Missionteens.Com
Salvation Army (Arc)	Adults	6 To 9 Mo.	800-728-7825	Satruck.Org
Victory Outreach	Adults	1 Year	708-850-1200 773-224-0201 773-568-1785 815-961-8583 (708-749-	Victoryoutreach.Org

			9080 Hispanic)	
Chicago Dream Center	Women	1 Year	773-384-2200	Chicago-dreamcenter.Org

Indiana
(call the centers to confirm)

Name Of Christian Rehab	Gender	Program Length	Contact	Website Address
Life Challenge / Teen Challenge	Adults And Teen Programs	1 Year	417-581-2181	Teenchallengeusa.Com
Salvation Army (Arc)	Adults	6 To 9 Mo.	800-728-7825	Satruck.Org
House Of Hope	Adults	Long-Term	812-446-1717	Missionteens.Com
Wheeler Mission Ministries	Adults		(317) 635-3575	Wheelermission.Org/

Iowa

Name Of Christian Rehab	Gender	Program Length	Contact	Website Address
Life Challenge / Teen Challenge	Adults And Teen Programs	1 Year	417-581-2181	Teenchallengeusa.Com
Proverbs Ministries	Men	1 Year	319-389-8992	Proverbsministries.Org

Salvation Army (Arc)	Adults	6 To 9 Mo.	800-728-7825	Satruck.Org
Victory Outreach	Adults	1 Year	515-244-2784	Victoryoutreach.Org
Midwest Mbtc	Adults	Long-Term	563-547-3286	Missionteens.Com

Illinois
(call the centers to confirm)

Name Of Christian Rehab	Gender	Program Length	Contact	Website Address
Life Challenge / Teen Challenge	Adults And Teen Programs	1 Year	417-581-2181	Teenchallengeusa.Com
Reformers Unanimous Residential	Adults	6 Months	866-733-6768	Ruhomes.Org
First Fruits	Adults	Long-Term	618-498-3560	Missionteens.Com
Salvation Army (Arc)	Adults	6 To 9 Mo.	800-728-7825	Satruck.Org
Victory Outreach	Adults	1 Year	708-850-1200 773-224-0201 773-568-1785 815-961-8583 (708-749-9080 Hispanic)	Victoryoutreach.Org
Chicago Dream Center	Women	1 Year	773-384-2200	Chicago-dreamcenter.Org

Indiana
(call the centers to confirm)

Name Of Christian Rehab	Gender	Program Length	Contact	Website Address
Life Challenge / Teen Challenge	Adults And Teen Programs	1 Year	417-581-2181	Teenchallengeusa.Com
Salvation Army (Arc)	Adults	6 To 9 Mo.	800-728-7825	Satruck.Org
House Of Hope	Adults	Long-Term	812-446-1717	Missionteens.Com
Wheeler Mission Ministries	Adults		(317) 635-3575	Wheelermission.Org/

Iowa

Name Of Christian Rehab	Gender	Program Length	Contact	Website Address
Life Challenge / Teen Challenge	Adults And Teen Programs	1 Year	417-581-2181	Teenchallengeusa.Com
Proverbs Ministries	Men	1 Year	319-389-8992	Proverbsministries.Org
Salvation Army (Arc)	Adults	6 To 9 Mo.	800-728-7825	Satruck.Org
Victory Outreach	Adults	1 Year	515-244-2784	Victoryoutreach.Org
Midwest Mbtc	Adults	Long-Term	563-547-3286	Missionteens.Com

Kansas
(call the centers to confirm)

Name Of Christian Rehab	Gender	Program Length	Contact	Website Address
Life Challenge / Teen Challenge	Adults And Teen Programs	1 Year	417-581-2181	Teenchallengeusa.Com
Salvation Army (Arc)	Adults	6 To 9 Mo.	800-728-7825	Satruck.Org

Kentucky

Name Of Christian Rehab	Gender	Program Length	Contact	Website Address
Life Challenge /Teen Challenge	Adults And Teen Programs	1 Year	417-581-2181	Teenchallengeusa.Com
City Of Hope	Men	1 Year	502-413-0102 Ext.1803	Mycityofhope.Com
Salvation Army (Arc)	Adults	6 To 9 Mo.	800-728-7825	Satruck.Org
M.B.T.C	Adults		606-349-7607	Missionteens.Com
Hope Center	Women	Long-Term	859-252-2002	Hopectr.Org
Hope Center	Men	Long-Term	859-225-4631	Hopectr.Org

Louisiana
(call the centers to confirm)

Name Of Christian Rehab	Gender	Program Length	Contact	Website Address
Life Challenge / Teen Challenge	Adults And Teen Programs	1 Year	417-581-2181	Teenchallengeusa.Com
Fresh Start Ministry	Men	Long Term	318-435-7061	Freshstartministry.Com
Freedom Challenge	Men		(318) 669-4826	
All The Way House	Adults	1 Year	225-287-9412 225-775-4321	Allthewayhouse.Org
Salvation Army (Arc)	Adults	6 To 9 Mo.	800-728-7825	Satruck.Org
Evangel House	Girls		800-924-4012	Evangelhouse.Com
Mercy Ministries	Women	Long Term	615-831-6987	Mercyministries.Org

Maine

Name Of Christian Rehab	Gender	Program Length	Contact	Website Address
Life Challenge / Teen Challenge	Adults And Teen Programs	1 Year	417-581-2181	Teenchallengeusa.Com
Seven Oaks Training Center	Men		207-991-9555	
Salvation Army (Arc)	Adults	6 To 9 Mo.	800-728-7825	Satruck.Org

Maryland
(call the centers to confirm)

Name Of Christian Rehab	Gender	Program Length	Contact	Website Address
Life Challenge / Teen Challenge	Adults And Teen Programs	1 Year	417-581-2181	Teenchallengeusa.Com
New Life For Girls	Adults	1 Year	(410) 848-1360	Newlifeforgirls.Org
Salvation Army (Arc)	Adults	6 To 9 Mo.	800-728-7825	Satruck.Org
Victory Outreach	Adults	1 Year	443-759-5735 240 619-4622	Victoryoutreach.Org
Helping Up Mission	Adults	12-Month	410-675-7500	Helpingupmission.Org

Massachusetts

Name Of Christian Rehab	Gender	Program Length	Contact	Website Address
Life Challenge/ Teen Challenge	Adults And Teen Programs	1 Year	417-581-2181	Teenchallengeusa.Com
Salvation Army (Arc)	Adults	6 To 9 Mo.	800-728-7825	Satruck.Org
Bridge House			781 593 3898	

Michigan

Name Of Christian Rehab	Gender	Program Length	Contact	Website Address
Life Challenge /Teen Challenge	Adults And Teen Programs	1 Year	417-581-2181	Teenchallengeusa.Com
Mission Bible Training Center	Adults	Long-Term	906-625-6247	Missionteens.Com
Alcohol Chemical Treatment Series (Acts)	Adults	24 Weeks	248-879-2447	Faith-Apostolic.Com
Salvation Army (Arc)	Adults	6 To 9 Mo.	800-728-7825	Satruck.Org
Kalamazoo Gospel Mission	Adults	Long-Term	269-345-2974	
Grace Discipleship	Young Men (Ages 18 - 35)		586-405-1796	
Pathway To Freedom			586 783-6939	
The New Life In Christ Program	Men		616-451-0236 X25	Lifeonthestreet.Org
Victory Outreach	Adults	1 Year	313-975-6413	Victoryoutreach.Org

Minnesota
(call the centers to confirm)

Name Of Christian Rehab	Gender	Program Length	Contact	Website Address
Life Challenge/ Teen Challenge	Adults And Teen Programs	1 Year	417-581-2181	Teenchallengeusa.Com

| Metro Hope | Men/Women | | 612-721-9415 | Metrohope.Org |

Mississippi
(call the centers to confirm)

Name Of Christian Rehab	Gender	Program Length	Contact	Website Address
Life Challenge / Teen Challenge	Adults And Teen Programs	1 Year	417-581-2181	Teenchallengeusa.Com
Mercy House Ministries	Men	1 Year	601-858-2256	
Home Of Grace	Adults		228-826-5283	Homeofgrace.Org
Salvation Army (Arc)	Adults	6 To 9 Mo.	800-728-7825	Satruck.Org

Missouri

Name Of Christian Rehab	Gender	Program Length	Contact	Website Address
Life Challenge / Teen Challenge	Adults And Teen Programs	1 Year	417-581-2181	Teenchallengeusa.Com
Genesis Men's Home	Men	1 Year	314-381-0700	Stldreamcenter.Org/Outreaches/Genesis-Mens-Home
Dream Center	Men & Women's Programs	Long-term	417-678-6909	
Heartland	Men		(660) 284-6212	
Mercy Ministries	Women	Long-term	615-831-6987	Mercyministries.Org

Hillcrest	Women/Kid		816-781-8988 816-461-0468	Hillcresttransitional-housing.Org

Montana
(call the centers to confirm)

Name Of Christian Rehab	Gender	Program Length	Contact	Website Address
Life Challenge /Teen Challenge	Adults And Teen Programs	1 Year	417-581-2181	Teenchal-lengeusa.Com
Great Falls Christian Discipleship Program	Adults		406-761-2653	Greatfallsres-cuemission.Com

Nebraska

Name Of Christian Rehab	Gender	Program Length	Contract	Website Address
Life Challenge / Teen Challenge	Adults And Teen Programs	1 Year	417-581-2181	Teenchal-lengeusa.Com

New Hampshire
(call the centers to confirm)

Name Of Christian Rehab	Gender	Program Length	Contact	Website Address
Life Challenge / Teen Challenge	Adults And Teen Programs	1 Year	417-581-2181	Teenchal-lengeusa.Com
His Mansion		1 Year	603-464-5555	Hismansion.Com

Name Of Christian Rehab	Gender	Program Length	Contact	Website Address
New Life Home	Women And Children		603-624-8444	Newlifehome.Org
Salvation Army (Arc)	Adults	6 To 9 Mo.	800-728-7825	Satruck.Org

New Jersey
(call the centers to confirm)

Name Of Christian Rehab	Gender	Program Length	Contact	Website Address
Life Challenge / Teen Challenge	Adults And Teen Programs	1 Year	417-581-2181	Teenchallengeusa.Com
Mbtc	Adults	Long-Term	856-691-9855	Missionteens.Com
The Empowerment Resurrection Center	Adults	Long-Term	856-575-0500	Erc-Njdrugrehab.Org
Salvation Army (Arc)	Adults	6 To 9 Mo.	800-728-7825	Satruck.Org
Victory Outreach	Adults	1 Year	856-361-7243 973-531-8024	Victoryoutreach.Org
Market Street Mission		10 Month	(973) 538-0431	Marketstreet.Org
U-Turn For Christ	Men	2 Or 10 Month	(908) 420-9586	
Good News Home For Women	Women	9 To 18 Month	908-806-4220	Goodnews-home.Org
America's Keswick	Adults	120-Day	732-350-1187 X 46	

New Mexico
(call the centers to confirm)

Name Of Christian Rehab	Gender	Program Length	Contact	Website Address
Life Challenge / Teen Challenge	Adults And Teen Programs	1 Year	417-581-2181	Teenchallengeusa.Com
U-Turn For Christ		2 Months +	505-903-8194	Uturnforchrist.Com

New York

Name Of Christian Rehab	Gender	Program Length	Contact	Website Address
Buffalo Adult And Teen Challenge	Men	1 Year	716-855-0602	Newyorkteenchallenge.Com
Life Challenge / Teen Challenge	Adults And Teen Programs	1 Year	417-581-2181	Teenchallengeusa.Com
New Life For Girls	Adults	1 Year	(718) 731-2752	Newlifeforgirls.Org
Freedom Village	Teens		(607)243-8126	Freedomvillageusa.Com
Anchor House	Adults	1 Year	718-771-0760	Anchorhousenyc.Org
Tlc	Men	6 Months	845-384-6511	Tlc911.Org
Walter Hoving Home	Women	6 Mo. To 1 Year	(845) 424-3674	
Victory Outreach	Adults	1 Year	718-393-8321 718-669-	Victoryoutreach.Org

			1927 646-606-6727 (718-768-3638 Hispanic)	
Life Change	Young Women Aged 16 – 25		845-586-4848	
Salvation Army (Arc)	Adults	6 To 9 Mo.	800-728-7825	Satruck.Org

North Carolina
(call the centers to confirm)

Name Of Christian Rehab	Gender	Program Length	Contact	Website Address
Life Challenge / Teen Challenge	Adults And Teen Programs	1 Year	417-581-2181	Teenchallengeusa.Com
Hebron Colony		60 Days	828-963-4842	Hebroncolony.Org
Bethel Colony	Men	65 Days	828-754-3781 828-754-9987	Bethelcolony.Org
Living Free Ministries	Men	9 Months	336-376-5066	Livingfreeministries.Net
In Him Ministries	Men	1 Year	910-322-7796	Inhimministriesinc.Com
House Of Prayer		3 To 6 Months	336-882-1026	Alcoholicshome.Org
Charlotte Rescue Mission & Rebound & Dove's Nest	Adults		704-333-Hope (4673)	Charlotterescuemission.Org

Armor of God

Name	Gender	Program Length	Contact	Website
The Victory Program	Adults	12-Month	919-688-9641	Durhamrescuemission.Org
Hosea House God Did It Recovery Home For Women	Women		919-304-6885 252-473-9324	
Freedom House	Women & Children	1 Year	336-286-7622	Helpfreedomhouse.Org
Jacob House & Zadok House	Men		919-580-9276 919-735-8094	
Safe Harbor Rescue Mission	Women	1 Year	828-326-7233	Safeharborrescuemission.Org
Charlotte Rescue Mission			704-334-4635	Charlotterescuemission.Org
Salvation Army (Arc)	Adults	6 To 9 Mo.	800-728-7825	Satruck.Org
Freedom Farm Ministries	Men		828-964-2914	Freedomfarmministries.Org

North Dakota
(call the centers to confirm)

Name Of Christian Rehab	Gender	Program Length	Contact	Website Address
Life Challenge / Teen Challenge	Adults And Teen Programs	1 Year	417-581-2181	Teenchallengeusa.Com

Ohio
(call the centers to confirm)

Name Of Christian Rehab	Gender	Program Length	Contact	Website Address
Life Challenge / Teen Challenge	Adults And Teen Programs	1 Year	417-581-2181	Teenchallengeusa.Com
Midwest Dream Center	Adults	1 Year	937-544-5908	Midwestdreamcenter.Com
Salvation Army (Arc)	Adults	6 To 9 Mo.	800-728-7825	Satruck.Org
Changing Lives Now	Men/Women		937-323-6396	Changinglivesnow.Org
Good Samaritan's Inn	Men	6-Month	513-896-5354	Christian-Drug-Alcohol-Treatment-Center.Org
Victory Outreach	Adults	1 Year	216-961-5121	Victoryoutreach.Org
(Crc) Cincinnati Restoration Church	Men/Women	9 Months	513-333-0212 877-803-5578	Cintirestoration.Org
City Gospel Mission	Men/Women	1 Year	513-241-5525	Citygospelmission.Org

Oklahoma

Name Of Christian Rehab	Gender	Program Length	Contact	Website Address
Adult Teen Challenge	Men / Women	1 Year	405-600-1920	Okteenchallenge.Com
Rob's Ranch	Men	90 Days	405-253-3838	Robsranch.Org

Salvation Army (Arc)	Adults	6 To 9 Mo.	800-728-7825	Satruck.Org
Clay Crossing		4 Mo.	866-374-1220	Claycrossing.Com
Renewal			866-428-8690	Renewalchristiancare.Com

Oregon
(call the centers to confirm)

Name Of Christian Rehab	Gender	Program Length	Contact	Website Address
Teen Challenge	Adults	1 Year	417-862-6969	Teenchallengeusa.Com
Northwest Mbtc	Adults	8 months	503-289-7758	Missionteens.Com
U Turn For Christ			541-291-3040 541-292-9388	Uturnforchristoregon.Org
Salvation Army (Arc)	Adults	6 To 9 Mo.	800-728-7825	Satruck.Org

Pennsylvania

Name Of Christian Rehab	Gender	Program Length	Contact	Website Address
Life Challenge / Teen Challenge	Adults And Teen	1 Year	417-581-2181	Teenchallengeusa.Com
New Life For Girls	Adults	1 Year	717-399-5435	Newlifeforgirls.Org
Salvation Army (Arc)	Adults	6 To 9 Mo.	800-728-7825	Satruck.Org
U Turn For Christ	Adults	2 Months +	717-376-4810	Uturnforchrist.Com
Victory Outreach	Adults	1 Year	215-426-5090	Victoryoutreach.Org
Refuge In Christ Recovery House	Adults		215-423-9290	

| Light Of Life | Adults | 9–18 Month | 412-258-6100 | Lightoflife.Org |

Rhode Island
(call the centers to confirm)

Name Of Christian Rehab	Gender	Program Length	Contact	Website Address
Life Challenge / Teen Challenge	Adults And Teen Programs	1 Year	417-581-2181	Teenchallengeusa.Com

South Carolina

Name Of Christian Rehab	Gender	Program Length	Contact	Website Address
Teen Challenge	Adults	1 Year	417-862-6969	Teenchallengeusa.Com
Grace Home	Women	2 Months	803-854-9809	Hebroncolony.Org
Faith Home	Adults	2 Months	864-223-0694 / 864-463-2363	Faithhomegwd.Net
Good Samaritan Colony	Men		843-634-6848	Goodsamaritancolony.Org
U Turn For Christ	Men	2 Months +	803-951-2197	Cclexington.Org/Ministries/U-Turn-For-Christ
Home With A Heart	Men		864-843-3058	Homewithaheart.Com
Haven Of Rest	Men/Women		864-226-6193	Havenofrest.Cc
Restoration Ranch			803-328-9427	Restorationranch.Org
Miracle Hill	Men/Women		(864) 268-4357	Miraclehill.Org

South Dakota
(call the centers to confirm)

Name Of Christian Rehab	Gender	Program Length	Contact	Website Address
Life Challenge / Teen Challenge	Adults And Teen Programs	1 Year	417-581-2181	Teenchallengeusa.Com

Tennessee

Name Of Christian Rehab	Gender	Program Length	Contact	Website Address
Life Challenge / Teen Challenge	Adults And Teen Programs	1 Year	417-581-2181	Teenchallengeusa.Com
U-Turn For Christ	Adults	2 Mo +	423-639-3720	Uturn4christtn.Com
Crossville Mbtc	Adults	Long Term	931-484-9935	Missionteens.Com
Miracle Lake	Adults		423-263-2583	Miraclelake.Org
Women At The Well Ministries	Women	18 Month	423-745-0010	The-womenatthewell.Com
Our Master's Camp	Men		423-447-2340	Ourmasterscamp.Org
Salvation Army (Arc)	Adults	6 To 9 Mo.	800-728-7825	Satruck.Org
Place Of Hope			931-388-9406	Placeofhopeinternational.Com
Mercy Ministries	Women	Long Term	615-831-6987	Mercyministries.Org

Texas
(call the centers to confirm)

Name Of Christian Rehab	Gender	Program Length	Contact	Website Address
Life Challenge / Teen Challenge	Adults And Teen Programs	1 Year	417-581-2181	Teenchallengeusa.Com
U-Turn For Christ	Men	2 Mo +	325-277-4784 325-944-8409	Uturn-forchristtexas.Com
Covenant With Christ	Women		(281)592-5007	
Northeast Texas Dream Center	Men	Long-Term	903-335-7188	Dreamcenter-texas.Com
East Texas Dream Center	Women	1 Year	281-601-6800	
House Of Destiny	Women		(936)274-5657	
Heartlight	Teens	9-12 Month	903-668-2173	Heartlightministries.Org
Shiloh Ministries	Men	1 Year	936-334-8616	Shilohmensministries.Com
Straight Way	Men	1 Year	979-532-5613	Straightway.Tc
East Texas Souls Harbor	Adults	1 Year	936-326-9850 936-652-3902	Easttexassoulsharbor.Org
Freedom Hill	Adults		979-337-9696	Freedomhill.Us
Strong Tower Ministries	Men		(855) 823-4546	

Armor of God

House Of Disciples	Men		(903) 553-0952	
Straight Street Ministries	Adults		972-291-2988	
Alvin South Coast Ministries	Men		(281) 585-9136	
Life Challenge Of Amarillo	Men		(806) 352-0385	
Victory Outreach	Adults	1 Year	817-759-9320 713-742-9000 915-307-8745 (512) 445-0478 (214) 826-4404 214-545-4130 214-317-7392 806-367-7033 210-533-7060 210-432-5150 (210) 226-3824 Hispanic)	Victoryoutreach.Org
Victory Family Center	Men		(713) 699-4357	
Men Of Nehemiah	Men		214-421-6705	Themenofnehemiah.Org
Salvation Army (Arc)	Adults	6 To 9 Mo.	800-728-7825	Satruck.Org

Victory Temple Ministries	Adults		Men: 817-626-1819 Women: 817-378-0921	Victorytemplerecovery.Org
Celebration Ministries	Adults	6 Months	512-332-2537	Celebration-bastrop.Org

Utah
(call the centers to confirm)

Name Of Christian Rehab	Gender	Program Length	Contact	Website Address
Life Challenge / Teen Challenge	Adults And Teen Programs	1 Year	417-581-2181	Teenchallengeusa.Com
One Way Ministry	Adults		435-201-2335	Ministryoneway.Webs.Com

Vermont

Name Of Christian Rehab	Gender	Program Length	Contact	Website Address
Life Challenge / Teen Challenge	Adults And Teen Programs	1 Year	417-581-2181	Teenchallengeusa.Com

Virginia
(call the centers to confirm)

Name Of Christian Rehab	Gender	Program Length	Contact	Website Address
Life Challenge / Teen Challenge	Adults And Teen Programs	1 Year	417-581-2181	Teenchallengeusa.Com
Elim Home	Men	2 Months	434-592-5629	Elimhome.Org
New Life For Youth	Men	Long-Term	(804) 448-2750	Newlifeforyouth.Com
New Life For Youth	Women	Long-Term	(804) 230-4485	Newlifeforyouth.Com

Washington

Name Of Christian Rehab	Gender	Program Length	Contact	Website Address
Life Challenge / Teen Challenge	Adults And Teen Programs	1 Year	417-581-2181	Teenchallengeusa.Com
Dream Center	Adults	1 Year	509-924-2630	Spokanedreamcenter.Org
Ruth's House Of Hope	Women		509-560-0714 509-476-Hope	Ruthshouseofhope.Org
Mountain Ministries	Men		360-430-7028	Mmrnw.Com
Mountain Ministries	Women / Children		360-560-6846	Mmrnw.Com
Praisealujah Discipleship	Adults	1 Year	206-251-8971	Praisealujah.Org

West Virginia
(call the centers to conform)

Name Of Christian Rehab	Gender	Program Length	Contact	Website Address
Life Challenge / Teen Challenge	Adults And Teen Programs	1 Year	417-581-2181	Teenchallengeusa.Com

Wisconsin

Name Of Christian Rehab	Gender	Program Length	Contact	Website Address
Life Challenge / Teen Challenge	Adults And Teen Programs	1 Year	417-581-2181	Teenchallengeusa.Com

Wyoming

Name Of Christian Rehab	Gender	Program Length	Contact	Website Address
Life Challenge / Teen Challenge	Adults And Teen Programs	1 Year	417-581-2181	Teenchallengeusa.Com
Salvation Army (Arc)	Adults	6 To 9 Mo.	800-728-7825	Satruck.Org

HOW TO CONTACT DEVINA?

Internet
- Herb Store: NaturalHealthEdu.com
- DevinaHCollier.com
- DivineNaturalSolutions.com
- Facebook.com/DevinaCollierNaturopath
- Facebook.com/DivineNaturalSolutions
- Youtube.com/c/DevinaCollierNaturopath

Speaking Request: Bible Studies, Events, T.V. and Radio Shows, Small Groups, Organizations or Churches.
Email: Info@DivineNaturalSolutions.com
Divine Natural Solutions - Private Healthcare Membership Association
P.O. Box 515 Flowery Branch, GA 30542

Other Books By Devina:
1. Rise and Shine 90 Day Devotional for Women with Evidence-Based Healing Foods
2. Hot Flashes, Memory Fog, Mood, and Fatigue
3. High Blood Pressure 28 Days Battle Plan
4. High Cholesterol 28 Days Battle Plan
5. Depression 28 Days Battle Plan
6. Anxiety and Stress 28 Days Battle Plan
7. Gut Restore 28 Days Battle Plan
8. Allergies 28 Days Battle Plan
9. Memory and Focus 28 Days Battle Plan

SPECIAL THANKS

To Dr. Annette Boone-Hicks for reviewing Armor Of God. Thank you for your review and for your prayers. When I read your review, I thanked God for it because it was precisely what this God-inspired book is about. God bless you and all of yours, dear women of God.

TheBooneClinicPC.com
Facebook.com/TheBooneClinicPC

To Angela Washington for the poems. You wrote those poems within a matter of minutes, and I didn't tell you what to write. I was astonished how accurate and inspirational they were. Thanks so much, strong woman of God for speaking into the lives of the readers.

Angelofwords.com
Facebook.com/AngelaWashingtonAngelofWords

To ReAnn Ring, an incredible multi-talented woman of God. Your creativity is incredible. It was a divine connection meeting you at The Christian View TV Talk Show. Truly, you are a blessing to the body of Christ. Thank you for the photography. They convey the Armor of God. I will forever be grateful. Thanks so much!

Images By ReAnn Ring: Front and Inside Cover
ReAnnRing.com
Facebook.com/ImagesByReAnn
Facebook.com/ReAnn.Ring

Evidence-Based Clinical Trials: Alternative Medicine

- [1] Randomised controlled trial of butterbur and cetirizine for treating seasonal allergic rhinitis. Published 19 January 2002. British Medical Journal. Andreas Schapowal, consultant in ear, nose, and throat medicine. Petasites Study Group.

- [2] Immunomodulation and Anti-Inflammatory Effects of Garlic Compounds. Journal of Immunology Research. 2015; 2015: 401630.

- [3] Prevention of allergic rhinitis by ginger and the molecular basis of immunosuppression by 6-gingerol through T cell inactivation. J Nutr Biochem. 2016 Jan;27:112-22.

- [4] The effects of spirulina on allergic rhinitis. European Archives of Oto-Rhino-Laryngology. October 2008, Volume 265, Issue 10, pp 1219–1223. Cemal CingiEmail author-Meltem Conk-DalayHamdi CakliCengiz Bal.

- [5] Moringa oleifera: a food plant with multiple medicinal uses. Farooq Anwar, Sajid Latif, Muhammad Ashraf, Anwarul Hassan Gilani.

- [6] Randomised, Double-Blind Study of Freeze-Dried Urtica dioica in the Treatment of Allergic Rhinitis. Paul Mittman. Georg Thieme Verlag Stuttgart New York.

- [7] Immunomodulatory effects of curcumin in allergy. Mol Nutr Food Res. 2008 Sep;52(9). Kurup VP, Barrios CS.

- [8] Medically reviewed by Debra Rose Wilson, PhD, MSN, RN, IBCLC, AHN-BC, CHT on April 26, 2017 — Written by Ana Gotter 5 Essential Oils for Headaches and Migraines. Healthline.com

- [9] Sasannejad P. Saeedi M.a. Shoeibi A. Gorji A. Abbasi M. Foroughipour M. Lavender Essential Oil in the Treatment of Migraine Headache: A Placebo-Controlled Clinical

Trial. European Neurology. 2012;67:288–291.

- [10] Sicuteri, Federigo; Fusco, Bruno M.; Marabini, Simone; Campagnolo, Valter; Maggi, Carlo Alberto; Geppetti, Pierangelo; Fanciullacci, Marcello. Beneficial Effect of Capsaicin Application to the Nasal Mucosa in Cluster Headache. Clinical Journal of Pain: March 1989.

- [11] Analyzing the interaction of a herbal compound Andrographolide from Andrographis paniculata as a folklore against swine flu (H1N1). Chandrabhan Seniya, Shilpi Shrivastava, Sanjay Kumar Singh, Ghulam Jilani Khan. Asian Pacific Journal of Tropical Disease. Volume 4, Supplement 2, September 2014, Pages S624-S630. Sciencedirect.com/science/article/pii/S2222180814606927

- [12] Harnessing the medicinal properties of Andrographis paniculata for diseases and beyond: a review of its phytochemistry and pharmacology. Agbonlahor Okhuarobo, Joyce Ehizogie Falodun, Osayemwenre Erharuyi, Vincent Imieje, Abiodun Falodun, and Peter Langer. Asian Pac J Trop Dis. 2014 Jun; 4(3): 213-222.
- [13] Andrographis Overview. Webmd.com/vitamins-supplements/ingredientmono-973-andrographis.aspx?activeingredientid=973&activeingredientname=andrographis
- [14] Comparing the effects of ginger and metoclopramide on the treatment of pregnancy nausea. Pak J Biol Sci. 2011 Aug 15;14(16):817-20. Mohammadbeigi R, Shahgeibi S, Soufizadeh N, Rezaiie M, Farhadifar F.

- [15] Foeniculum vulgare: A comprehensive review of its traditional use, phytochemistry, pharmacology, and safety. Arabian Journal of Chemistry. Volume 9, Supplement 2, Nov. 2016, Pages S1574-S1583. Manzoor A.Rather, Bilal A.Dar, Shahnawaz N.Sofi, Bilal A.Bhat, Mushtaq A.Qurishi.
- [16] The Effect of Aromatherapy Inhalation on Nausea and Vomiting in Early Pregnancy: A Pilot Randomised Controlled Trial. Journal of Natural Sciences Research www.iiste.org. ISSN 2224-3186 (Paper) ISSN 2225-0921 (Online). Vol.3, No.5, 2013. Rania Mahmoud Abdel Ghani, Adlia Tawfik Ahmed Ibrahim.
- [17] Nutrients. 2015 Sep; 7(9): 7729–7748. Antibacterial Effects of Cinnamon: From Farm to Food, Cosmetic and Pharmaceutical Industries. Seyed Fazel Nabavi, Arianna Di Lorenzo, Morteza Izadi, Eduardo Sobarzo-Sánchez, Maria Daglia, and Seyed Mohammad Nabavi.

- [18] Iran Red Crescent Med J. 2014 Mar; 16(3). The Effect of Lemon Inhalation Aromatherapy on Nausea and Vomiting of Pregnancy: A Double-Blinded, Randomised, Controlled Clinical Trial. Parisa Yavari kia, Farzaneh Safajou, Mahnaz Shahnazi, and Hossein Nazemiyeh.
- [19] J Holist Nurs. 2012 Jun;30(2):90-104. Examination of the effectiveness of peppermint aromatherapy on nausea in women post C-section. Lane B, Cannella K, Bowen C, Copelan D, Nteff G, Barnes K, Poudevigne M, Lawson J.
- [20] Ecancermedicalscience. 2013; 7: 290. Antiemetic activity of volatile oil from Mentha spicata and Mentha × piperita in chemotherapy-induced nausea and vomiting. Z Tayarani-Najaran, E Talasaz-Firoozi, R Nasiri, N Jalali, and MK Hassanzadeh.
- [21] Middle East J Dig Dis. 2013 Oct; 5(4): 217–222. Cumin Extract for Symptom

Control in Patients with Irritable Bowel Syndrome: A Case Series. Shahram Agah, Amir Mehdi Taleb, Reyhane Moeini, Narjes Gorji, and Hajar Nikbakht.
- [22] Clove: A champion spice. Parle, Milind & Deepa, Khanna. (2010). International Journal of Research in Ayurveda and Pharmacy. 2.
- [23] World J Gastroenterol. 2011 Jan 7; 17(1): 105–110. Effect of ginger on gastric motility and symptoms of functional dyspepsia
- [24] Syst Rev. 2014; 3: 71. Jun 28. Efficacy of turmeric in the treatment of digestive disorders: a systematic review and meta-analysis protocol. Kednapa Thavorn, Muhammad M Mamdani, and Sharon E Straus.
- [25] Nasrin Fazel. Akbar Pejhan. Mohsen Taghizadeh. Yaser Tabarraei. Nasrin Sharifi. Effects of Anethum graveolens L. (Dill) essential oil on the intensity of retained intestinal gas, flatulence and pain after cesarean

section: A randomised, double-blind placebo-controlled trial. Journal of Herbal Medicine. Volume 8, June 2017, Pages 8-13.

- [26] Iran Red Crescent Med J. 2016 Apr; 18(4): Prevention and Treatment of Flatulence From a Traditional Persian Medicine Perspective. Bagher Larijani, Mohammad Medhi Esfahani, Maryam Moghimi, Mohammad Reza Shams Ardakani, Mansoor Keshavarz, Gholamreza Kordafshari, Esmaiel Nazem, Shirin Hasani Ranjbar, Hoorieh Mohammadi Kenari, and Arman Zargaran.

- [27] Middle East J Dig Dis. 2013 Oct; 5(4): 217–222. Cumin Extract for Symptom Control in Patients with Irritable Bowel Syndrome: A Case Series. Shahram Agah, Amir Mehdi Taleb, Reyhane Moeini, Narjes Gorji, and Hajar Nikbakht.

- [28] Clove: A champion spice. Flatulence Facts & Phytonutrient Cliches. A bird Eye view. Parle, Milind & Deepa, Khanna. (2010). International Journal of Research in Ayurveda and Pharmacy. 2.
- [29] Arabian Journal of Chemistry. Volume 9, Supplement 2, November 2016, Pages S1574-S1583. Foeniculum vulgare: A comprehensive review of its traditional use, phytochemistry, pharmacology, and safety. Manzoor A. Rathera, Bila A. Dara, Shahnawaz N. Sofi, Bilal A. Bhat, Mushtaq A. Qurishi.
- [30] A comparative study of dimethicone and supermint anti-flatulence effects on reducing flatulence in patients with irritable bowel syndrome. Nasiri, A.A. & Pakmehr, M & Shahdadi, Hosien & Balouchi, Abbas & Sepehri, Zahra & Ghalenov, A.R. (2016). 8. 97-101.

- [31] Res Pharm Sci. 2011 Jan-Jun; 6(1): 13–21. Effects of extract and essential oil of Rosmarinus officinalis L. on TNBS-induced colitis in rats. M. Minaiyan, A. R. Ghannadi, M. Afsharipour, and P. Mahzouni.
- [32] Eating Well During and After Your Cancer Treatment. Memorial Sloan Kettering Cancer Center. Mskcc.org/cancer-care/patient-education/eating-well-during-and-after-your-treatment
- [33] Why you should eat your collard greens. October 2016 By Megan Ware. Reviewed by Deborah Weatherspoon, PhD, RN, CRNA.
- [34] Kiwifruit promotes laxation in the elderly. Asia Pac J Clin Nutr. 2002;11(2):164-8. Rush EC, Patel M, Plank LD, Ferguson LR.
- [35] Increasing dietary fiber intake in terms of kiwifruit improves constipation in Chinese patients. Chan, A. O., et al. World J Gastroenterol. 13(35):4771-4775, 2007.

- [36] Stacewicz-Sapuntzakis, M., et al. Chemical composition and potential health effects of prunes: a functional food? Crit Rev Food Sci Nutr. 41(4):251-286, 2001.

- [37] Randomized, double-blind, placebo-controlled trial of Ficus carica paste for the management of functional constipation. Baek HI, Ha KC, Kim HM, Choi EK, Park EO, Park BH, Yang HJ, Kim MJ, Kang HJ, Chae SW. Asia Pac J Clin Nutr. 2016;25(3):487-96.

- [38] Standardized senna extract generally produced a bowel movement within six to 12 hours of its ingestion (without causing cramping). English, J. Research preview for the new millennium. Vitamin Research News. Jan 2000.

- [39] Psyllium (Plantago ovata). Alternative Medicine Review 2002, 7(2):155-159.

- [40] Mitochondrial Dysfunction and Chronic Fatigue Syndromes:Issues in Clinical Care Th. Bihari Singh, Kh.Robindro Singh. IOSR Journal of Dental and Medical Sciences (IOSR-JDMS). e-ISSN: 2279-0853, p-ISSN: 2279-0861.Volume 13, Issue 5 Ver. V. (May. 2014), PP 30-33. www.iosrjournals.org

- [41] Indian J Psychol Med. 2012 Jul-Sep; 34(3): 255–262. A Prospective, Randomised Double-Blind, Placebo-Controlled Study of Safety and Efficacy of a High-Concentration Full-Spectrum Extract of Ashwagandha Root in Reducing Stress and Anxiety in Adults. K. Chandrasekhar, Jyoti Kapoor, and Sridhar Anishetty.

- [42] Nutr J. 2010; 9: 55. High cacao polyphenol rich chocolate may reduce the burden of the symptoms in chronic fatigue syndrome.

- [43] Effect of Ginkgo and Cistanche Against Fatigue Symptoms (GkoCist). U.S. National

Library of Medicine. Sinphar Pharmaceutical Co., Ltd. SPRIM China (Shanghai) Consulting Co., LTD. and Fudan University.

- [44] Black CD, O'Connor PJ. Acute effects of dietary ginger on muscle pain induced by eccentric exercise. Phyther Res [Internet]. 2010 Nov [cited 2018 Mar 27];24(11):1620–6.

- [45] Terry R, Posadzki P, Watson LK, Ernst E. The Use of Ginger (Zingiber officinale) for the Treatment of Pain: A Systematic Review of Clinical Trials. Pain Med [Internet]. 2011 Dec 1 [cited 2018 Mar 27];12(12):1808–18.

- [46] Daily JW, Yang M, Park S. Efficacy of Turmeric Extracts and Curcumin for Alleviating the Symptoms of Joint Arthritis: A Systematic Review and Meta-Analysis of Randomised Clinical Trials. J Med Food [Internet]. 2016 Aug [cited 2018 Mar 27];19(8):717–29.

- [47] Kyokong, O., Charuluxananan, S., Muangmingsuk, V., Rodanant, O., Subornsug, K., & Punyasang, W. (2002). Efficacy of chamomile-extract spray for prevention of postoperative sore throat. Journal of the Medical Association of Thailand, 85, Suppl 1:S180-S18.

- [48] Jung HL, Kwak HE, Kim SS, Kim YC, Lee C Do, Byurn HK, et al. Effects of Panax ginseng Supplementation on Muscle Damage and Inflammation after Uphill Treadmill Running in Humans. Am J Chin Med [Internet]. 2011 Jan [cited 2018 Mar 27];39(3):441–50.

- [49] Mashhadi NS, Ghiasvand R, Askari G, Feizi A, Hariri M, Darvishi L, et al. Influence of ginger and cinnamon intake on inflammation and muscle soreness endued by exercise in Iranian female athletes. Int J Prev Med [Internet]. 2013 Apr [cited 2018 Mar 27];4(Suppl 1):S11-5.

- [50] Mathias, B. J., Dillingham, T. R., Zeigler, D. N., Chang, A. S., & Belandres, P. V. (1995). Topical capsaicin for chronic neck pain. A pilot study. American Journal of Physical Medicine & Rehabilitation, 74, 39-44.

- [51] Deal, C. L., Schnitzer, T. J., Lipstein, E., Seibold, J. R., Stevens, R. M., Levy, M. D., et al. (1991). Treatment of arthritis with topical capsaicin: A double-blind trial. Clinical Therapeutics, 13, 383-395.

- [52] Apan, A., Buyukkocak, U., Ozcan, S., Sari, E., & Basar, H. (2004). Postoperative magnesium sulphate infusion reduces analgesic requirements in spinal anaesthesia. European Journal of Anaesthesiology, 21, 766-769.

- [53] Crosby, V., Wilcock, A., & Corcoran, R. (2000). The safety and efficacy of a single dose (500 mg or 1 g) of intravenous magnesium sulfate in neuropathic pain poorly responsive to strong opioid analgesics in patients with cancer. Journal of Pain & Symptom.

- [54] Chrubasik S, Eisenberg E, Balan E, Weinberger T, Luzzati R, Conradt C. Treatment of low back pain exacerbations with willow bark extract: a randomised double-blind study. Am J Med [Internet]. 2000 Jul [cited 2018 Mar 27];109(1):9–14.

- [55] Chrubasik S, Künzel O, Model A, Conradt C, Black A. Treatment of low back pain with a herbal or synthetic anti-rheumatic: a randomised controlled study. Willow bark extract for low back pain. Rheumatology (Oxford) [Internet]. 2001 Dec [cited 2018 Mar 27];40(12):1388–93.

- [56] Fiebich BL, Chrubasik S. Effects of an ethanolic Salix extract on the release of selected inflammatory mediators in vitro.

Phytomedicine [Internet]. 2004 Jan [cited 2018 Mar 27];11(2–3):135–8.

- [57] Meamarbashi A, Abbasian M. The effects of Cinnamon and Indomethacin in prevention of Delayed Onset Muscle Soreness (DOMS). Proceedings of International Conference on Medical & Health Sciences; 22-24 May 2013; Kota Bharu, Malaysia.

- [58] Journal of Affective Disorders. Volume 78, Issue 2, February 2004, Pages 101-110. Clinical efficacy of kava extract WS® 1490 in sleep disturbances associated with anxiety disorders: Results of a multicenter, randomised, placebo-controlled, double-blind clinical trial. Siegfried Lehrl.

- [59] The Journal of Alternative and Complementary Medicine. Vol 11, Number 4, 2005, pp. 631–637. © Mary Ann Liebert, Inc. A Single-Blinded, Randomised Pilot Study

Evaluating the Aroma. of Lavandula augustifolia as a Treatment for Mild Insomnia.

- [60] Neuropsychiatr Dis Treat. 2016; 12: 1715–1723. Published online 2016 Jul 11. A meta-analysis on the efficacy and safety of St John's wort extract in depression therapy in comparison with selective serotonin reuptake inhibitors in adults. Yong-hua Cui, and Yi Zheng.

- [61] Am J Med. 2006 Dec; 119(12): 1005–1012. Valerian for Sleep: A Systematic Review and Meta-Analysis. Stephen Bent, MD, Amy Padula, MS, Dan Moore, PhD, Michael Patterson, MS, and Wolf Mehling, MD.

- [62] Jerome Sarris. Alexander Panossian. Isaac Schweitzer. Con Stough. Andrew Scholey. Herbal medicine for depression, anxiety and insomnia: A review of psychopharmacology and clinical evidence. European Neuropsychopharmacology. Volume

21, Issue 12, December 2011, Pages 841-860.

- [63] Med J Nutrition Metab. 2011 Dec; 4(3): 211–218. Pilot trial of Melissa officinalis L. leaf extract in the treatment of volunteers suffering from mild-to-moderate anxiety disorders and sleep disturbances. Julien Cases, Alvin Ibarra, Nicolas Feuillère, Marc Roller, and Samir G. Sukkar.

- [64] Preliminary examination of the efficacy and safety of a standardized chamomile extract for chronic primary insomnia: A randomised placebo-controlled pilot study. Suzanna M Zick, Benjamin D Wright, Ananda Sen and J Todd Arnedt. BMC Complementary and Alternative Medicine. The official journal of the International Society for Complementary Medicine Research (ISCMR)201111:78. 22 September 2011.

- [65] Phytother Res. 2011 Aug;25(8):1153-9. A double-blind, placebo-controlled investigation of the effects of Passiflora incarnata (passionflower) herbal tea on subjective sleep quality. Ngan A, Conduit R.
- [66] Phytomedicine. 2016 Dec 15;23(14):1735-1742. Long-term chamomile (Matricaria chamomilla L.) treatment for generalized anxiety disorder: A randomised clinical trial. Mao JJ, Xie SX, Keefe JR, Soeller I, Li QS, Amsterdam JD.
- [67] Mol Med Report. 2010 Nov 1; 3(6): 895–901. Chamomile: A herbal medicine of the past with bright future. Janmejai K Srivastava, Eswar Shankar, and Sanjay Gupta.
- [68] Journal of Affective Disorders. Volume 78, Issue 2, February 2004, Pages 101-110. Clinical efficacy of kava extract WS® 1490 in sleep disturbances associated with anxiety disorders: Results of a multicenter,

randomised, placebo-controlled, double-blind clinical trial. Siegfried Lehr.

- [69] Evid Based Complement Alternat Med. 2017; 2017: 5869315. The Effectiveness of Aromatherapy for Depressive Symptoms: A Systematic Review. Dalinda Isabel Sánchez-Vidaña, Shirley Pui-Ching Ngai, Wanjia He, Jason Ka-Wing Chow, Benson Wui-Man Lau, and Hector Wing-Hong Tsang.

- [70] Evid Based Complement Alternat Med. 2013. Lavender and the Nervous System. Peir Hossein Koulivand, Maryam Khaleghi Ghadiri, and Ali Gorji.

- [72] Evid Based Complement Alternat Med. 2017. The Effectiveness of Aromatherapy for Depressive Symptoms: A Systematic Review. Dalinda Isabel Sánchez-Vidaña, Shirley Pui-Ching Ngai, Wanjia He, Jason Ka-Wing Chow, Benson Wui-Man Lau, and Hector Wing-Hong Tsang.

- [73] McCaffrey R. Thomas DJ. Kinzelman AO. The effects of lavender and rosemary essential oils on test-taking anxiety among graduate nursing students. Holistic Nursing Practice - Journals. 2009 Mar-Apr;23(2):88-93

- [74] Proc Natl Acad Sci U S A. 1994 May 24; 91(11): 5148–5152. In vivo production of human factor VII in mice after intrasplenic implantation of primary fibroblasts transfected by receptor-mediated, adenovirus-augmented gene delivery. K Zatloukal, M Cotten, M Berger, W Schmidt, E Wagner, and M L Birnstiel.

- [75] Journal of Obstetrics and Gynaecology. Volume 38, 2018 - Issue 1. Effect of Foeniculum vulgare (fennel) on symptoms of depression and anxiety in postmenopausal women: a double-blind randomised controlled trial. Pages 121-126. 11 Sep 2017. Masumeh Ghazanfarpour, Fatemeh

Mohammadzadeh, Paymaneh shokrollahi, Talat Khadivzadeh, Mona Najaf Najafi, Hamidreza Hajirezaee and Maliheh Afiat.

- [76] The World Journal of Biological Psychiatry. Volume 10, 08 Dec 2009 - Issue 4-2. Ashwagandha for anxiety disorders. Chittaranjan Andrade, MD.

- [77] Med J Nutrition Metab. 2011 Dec; 4(3): 211–218. 2010 Dec 17. Pilot trial of Melissa officinalis L. leaf extract in the treatment of volunteers suffering from mild-to-moderate anxiety disorders and sleep disturbances. Julien Cases, Alvin Ibarra, Nicolas Feuillère, Marc Roller, and Samir G. Sukkar.

- [78] Altern Ther Health Med. 2003 Mar-Apr;9(2):74-8. An investigation into the efficacy of Scutellaria lateriflora in healthy volunteers. Wolfson P, and Hoffmann DL.

- [79] American Skullcap (Scutellaria lateriflora): a randomised, double-blind placebo-controlled crossover study of its effects on mood in healthy volunteers. Randomised controlled trial. Brock C, et al. Phytother Res. 2014. Brock C, Whitehouse J, Tewfik I, Towell T.

- [80] B. Raudenbush. T. Sears. R. Grayhem. I. Wilson.. Effects of peppermint and cinnamon odor administration on simulated driving alertness, mood and workload. Researchgate.net.

- [81] Hunter Groninger, M.D. Randall E. Schisler, M.D. Topical Capsaicin for Neuropathic Pain #255. Journal of Palliative Medicine. 2012 Aug; 15(8): 946–947.

- [82] Pharmacopsychiatry. 1997 Jan;30(1):1-5. Kava-kava extract WS 1490 versus placebo in anxiety disorders--a randomised placebo-controlled 25-week outpatient trial. Volz HP, Kieser M.

- [83] J Ethnopharmacol. 2003 Jan;84(1):91-4. The effects of aqueous extract of Lavandula angustifolia flowers in glutamate-induced neurotoxicity of cerebellar granular cell culture of rat pups. Büyükokuroğlu ME, Gepdiremen A, Hacimüftüoğlu A, Oktay M.

- [84] International Journal of Crude Drug Research. Volume 25, 1987 - Issue 1. Anticonvulsant Effects of Some Arab Medicinal Plants. A.-S. Abdul-Ghani, S. G. El-lati, A. I. Sacaan, M. S. Suleiman & R. M. Amin.

- [85] Effect of Rosmarinus officinalis L. Extract on the Seizure Induced by Picrotoxin in Mice. Pakistan Journal of Biological Sciences, 8: 1807-1811. M.R. Heidari, A. Assadipour, P. Rashid-farokhi, H. Assad and A. Mandegary. M.R. Heidari, A. Assadipour, P. Rashid-farokhi, H. Assad and A. Mandegary, 2005. DOI: 10.3923/pjbs.2005.1807.1811. URL:

https://scialert.net/abstract/?doi=pjbs.2005.1807.1811.

- [86] Brahmighritham, an Ayurvedic herbal formula for the control of epilepsy. J Ethnopharmacol. 1991 Jul;33(3):269-76. Shanmugasundaram ER, Akbar GK, Shanmugasundaram KR.

- [87] Effect of brahmi rasayan on the central nervous system. Journal of Ethnopharmacology. Volume 21, Issue 1, September 1987, Pages 65-74. Bina Shukia N.K. Khanna J.L. Godhwani.

- [88] Evaluation of the anticonvulsant effect of Centella asiatica (gotu kola) in pentylenetetrazol-induced seizures with respect to cholinergic neurotransmission. March 2010 Volume 17, Issue 3, Pages 332–335. Gopalreddygari Visweswari, Kanchi Siva Prasad, Pandanaboina Sahitya Chetan, Valluru Lokanatha, and Wudayagiri Rajendra.

- [89] An investigation into the efficacy of Scutellaria lateriflora in healthy volunteers. Altern Ther Health Med. 2003 Mar-Apr;9 (2): 74-8. Wolfson P, Hoffmann DL.
- [90] Altern Ther Health Med. 2012 Sep-Oct;18(5):44-9. Chamomile (Matricaria recutita) may provide antidepressant activity in anxious, depressed humans: an exploratory study. Amsterdam JD, Shults J, Soeller I, Mao JJ, Rockwell K, Newberg AB.
- [91] Modulatory Effects of Eschscholzia californica Alkaloids on Recombinant GABAA Receptors. Biochem Res Int. 2015; 2015: 617620. Milan Fedurco, Jana Gregorová, Kristýna Šebrlová, Jana Kantorová, Ondřej Peš, Roland Baur, Erwin Sigel, and Eva Táborská.
- [92] The Efficacy of Ginkgo for Elderly People with Dementia and Age-Associated Memory Impairment: New Results of a Randomised Clinical Trial. Journal of the American

Geriatrics Society. 27 April 2015. Martien C.J.M. van Dongen PhD, Erik van Rossum PhD, Alphons G.H. Kessels MD, Hilde J.G. Sielhorst RN, Paul G. Knipschild MD, PhD.

- [93] A Systematic Review and Meta-Analysis of Ginkgo biloba in Neuropsychiatric Disorders: From Ancient Tradition to Modern-Day Medicine. Evid Based Complement Alternat Med. 2013; 2013: 915691.
- [94] Kava for the treatment of generalized anxiety disorder (K-GAD): study protocol for a randomised controlled trial. BioMed Central 2015; 16: 493. Karen M. Savage, corresponding author Con K. Stough, Gerard J. Byrne, Andrew Scholey, Chad Bousman, Jenifer Murphy, Patricia Macdonald, Chao Suo, Matthew Hughes, Stuart Thomas, Rolf Teschke, Chengguo Xing, and Jerome Sarris.
- [95] World first clinical trial supports use of Kava to treat anxiety. Research finds Kava

significantly reduced the symptoms of people suffering anxiety. Journal of Clinical Psychopharmacology University of Melbourne. Dr Jerome Sarris. May 13, 2013.

- [96] Saffron (Crocus sativus L.) and major depressive disorder: a meta-analysis of randomised clinical trials. Hausenblas HA1, Saha D, Dubyak PJ, Anton SD. J Integr Med. 2013 Nov;11(6):377-83.
- [97] Saffron (Crocus sativus) for depression: a systematic review of clinical studies and examination of underlying antidepressant mechanisms of action. Lopresti AL, Drummond PD. Hum Psychopharmacol. 2014 Nov;29(6):517-27.
- [98] St John's wort for depression--an overview and meta-analysis of randomised clinical trials. K. Linde, G. Ramirez, C. D. Mulrow, A. Pauls, W. Weidenhammer, and D. Melchart. BMJ. 1996 Aug 3; 313(7052): 253–258.

- [99] St. John's Wort and Depression: In Depth. National Center for Complementary and Integrative Health. Jonathan R.T. Davidson, M.D., Duke University; David Mischoulon, M.D., Ph.D., Massachusetts General Hospital; and D. Craig Hopp, Ph.D., and David Shurtleff, Ph.D., NCCIH. Dec 2017.
- [100] Valerian and St. John's wort extract were effective in the treatment of depression and anxiety on the severity of premenstrual syndrome symptoms. Zahra Behboodi Moghadama, Elham Rezaei, Roghaieh Shirood Gholamia, Masomeh Kheirkhah, and Hamid Haghani. Journal of Traditional and Complementary Medicine. Volume 6, Issue 3, July 2016, Pages 309-315.
- [101] An Overview of Systematic Reviews of Ginkgo biloba Extracts for Mild Cognitive Impairment and Dementia. Hong-Feng Zhang, Li-Bo Huang, Yan-Biao Zhong, Qi-

Hui Zhou, Hui-Lin Wang, Guo-Qing Zheng, and Yan Lin. Frontier in Aging Neurosci 2016 Dec 6.

- [102] The effect of the essential oils of lavender and rosemary on the human short-term memory. O.V. Filiptsova, L.V. Gazzavi-Rogozina, I.A. Timoshyna, O.I. Naboka, Ye.V. Dyomina, and A.V. Ochkur. Alexandria Journal of Medicine. Volume 54, Issue 1, March 2018, Pages 41-44
- [103] The effect of the essential oils of lavender and rosemary on the human short-term memory. O.V. Filiptsova, L.V. Gazzavi-Rogozina, I.A. Timoshyna, O.I. Naboka, Ye.V. Dyomina, and A.V. Ochkur. Alexandria Journal of Medicine. Volume 54, Issue 1, March 2018, Pages 41-44.
- [104] Efficacy and Safety of Ashwagandha (Withania somnifera (L.) Dunal) Root Extract in Improving Memory and Cognitive Functions. Dnyanraj Choudhary, MD, Sauvik

Bhattacharyya, MPharm, PhD and Sekhar Bose, MPharm, PhD. Journal of Dietary Supplements. Volume 14, 2017 - Issue 6.

- [105] Antifatigue Effects of Panax ginseng C.A. Meyer: A Randomised, Double-Blind, Placebo-Controlled Trial. Hyeong-Geug Kim, Jung-Hyo Cho, Sa-Ra Yoo, Jin-Seok Lee, Jong-Min Han, Nam-Hun Lee, Yo-Chan Ahn, and Chang-Gue Son. PLOS One A Peer-Reviewed, Open Access Journal. 2013 Apr 17.

- [106] A double-blind, placebo-controlled study on the effects of Gotu Kola (Centella asiatica) on acoustic startle response in healthy subjects. Bradwejn J1, Zhou Y, Koszycki D, Shlik J. J Clin Psychopharmacol. 2000 Dec;20(6):680-4.

- [107] List of parasites of humans. From Wikipedia, the free encyclopedia. En.wikipedia.org/wiki/List_of_parasites_of_humans

- [108] Intestinal parasites. By SickKids hospital staff. Aboutkidshealth.ca/Article?contentid=815&language=English AboutKidsHealth.ca.

- [109] Parasitic Brain Infections. By John E. Greenlee, MD, Professor and Executive Vice Chair, Department of Neurology, University of Utah School of Medicine. Merck Sharp & Dohme Corp., a subsidiary of Merck & Co., Inc., Kenilworth, NJ, USA

- [110] Common Intestinal Parasites. Corry Jeb Kucik, LT, MC, Usn, Gary L. Martin, LCDR, MC, USN, And Brett V. Sortor, LCDR, MC, USN, Naval Hospital Jacksonville, Jacksonville, Florida. Am Fam Physician. 2004 Mar 1;69(5):1161-1169. Aaafp.org/afp/2004/0301/p1161.html

- [111] Signs and Symptoms of Parasites in Humans. Symptoms of parasites can arrive in humans after eating undercooked meat or touching pets. By UHN Staff. JAN 8, 2018. University Health News Daily.

- [112] What's to know about parasites? Feb 16, 2018. By Christian Nordqvist. Reviewed by Alana Biggers, MD, MPH. MedicalNewsToday. Medicalnewstoday.com/articles/220302.php

- [113] Probiotics for the Control of Parasites: An Overview. Marie-Agnès Travers, Isabelle Florent, Linda Kohl, and Philippe Grellier. J Parasitol Res. 2011; 2011: 610769. Ncbi.nlm.nih.gov/pmc/articles/PMC3182331

- [114] Lianet Monzote. Oswald Alarcón. William N. Setzer. Antiprotozoal Activity of Essential Oils: Review Article. Agriculturae Conspectus Scientifi cus. Vol. 77 (2012) No. 4 (167-175).

- [115] Colloidal silver. Health Search. 1(2), 1997. Doctors have successfully used silver for the treatment of intestinal parasites.

- [116] Black walnut is an anti-parasitic herb. Mindell, Earl R. The MSM Miracle. Keats Publishing, Lincolnwood, Illinois, USA, 1997:34-35.
- [117] Bunnag, D., et al. Southeast Asian J of Tropical Medicine and Public Health. 22:380-385, 1991. Cure rates of 90% - 100% were achieved with derivatives of qinghaosu (derived from Artemisia annua) for the treatment of falciparum malaria.
- [118] Chinese herb may have answer for malaria. Mediherb Monitor. June 1992, pp 2-3. Artemisia annua has a long history of use for the treatment of intestinal parasites in China. The active component has been identified as qinghaosu or artermisinine (a type of sesquiterpene lactone).
- [119] English, J. Candida yeast protection program. Part II: Freeing the body from candida and preventing recurrence. Vitamin

Research News. April 1999. The author advises that napthoquinones including lapachol in Pau D'Arco exert anti-parasitic effects.

- [120] Fife, Bruce. The Healing Miracles of Coconut Oil. Piccadilly Books, 2000.

- [121] Duez, P., et al. Journal of Ethnopharmacology. 34:235-246, 1991.

- [122] Mahmoud, M. R., et al. The effect of Nigella sativa oil against the liver damage induced by Schistosoma mansoni infection in mice. Journal of Ethnopharmacology. 79(1):1-11, 2002. Department of Pharmacology, Theodor Bilharz Research Institute, Imbaba, Giza, Egypt.

- [123] Force, M., et al. Inhibition of enteric parasites by emulsified oil of oregano in vivo. Phytotherapy Research. 14:213-214, 2000.

- [124] University of Maryland Medical Center. Wound healing and recovery from illness.

umm.edu/health/medical/altmed/supplement/glutamine.

- [125] Chen, G., et al. [Clinical observation of the protective effect of oral feeding of glutamine granules on intestinal mucous membrane]. Zhonghua Shao Shang Za Zhi. 17(4):210-211, 2001.

- [126] Probiotics and Prebiotics: Role in Clinical Disease States. Chien-Chang Chen, MD (Instructor, Research Fellow), W. Allan Walker, MD (Conrad Taff Professor of Nutrition and Pediatrics, Director) Advancesinpediatrics.org/article/S0065-3101(05)00002-2/fulltext

- [127] Webmd.com/digestive-disorders/tc/probiotics-topic-overview

- [128] Silk DB, Davis A, Vulevic J, Tzortzis G, Gibson GR. Clinical trial: the effects of a trans-galactooligosaccharide probiotic on fecal microbiota and symptoms in irritable bowel syndrome. Aliment Pharmacol Ther 2009; 29: 508-18.

- [129] Nobaek, S., et. Al. Alteration of intestinal microflora is associated with reduction in abdominal bloating and pain in patients with irritable bowel syndrome Microflora and IBS. American Journal of Gastroenterology, 2000, 95(5):1231-1238

- [130] Rolfe, R.D., et al. The role of probiotic cultures in the control of gastrointestinal health. Journal of Nutrition. 130(Supplement):396S-402S, 2000.

- [131] R. Balfour Sartor, M.D. Therapeutic manipulation of the enteric microflora in inflammatory bowel diseases: antibiotics, probiotics, and prebiotics. Division of Gastroenterology and Hepatology, Department of Medicine, Microbiology and Immunology, Center for Gastrointestinal Biology and Disease, University of North Carolina, Chapel

Hill, North Carolina, USA. Volume 126, Issue 6, May 2004, Pages 1620–1633

- [132] Effects of prebiotics on mineral metabolism. Katharina E Scholz-Ahrens, Gertjan Schaafsma, Ellen GHM van den Heuvel, Jürgen Schrezenmeir. The American Journal of Clinical Nutrition, Volume 73, Issue 2, 1 February 2001, Pages 459s–464s. Ajcn.org/content/73/2/459s.full?sid=d5a949dd-5ba7-4242-8536-f1d98a09cda3

- [133] Arabinogalactan supplement benefit and side effects. July 12, 2017 by Ray Sahelian, M.D. Raysahelian.com/arabinogalactan.html

- [134] Estrogen and Xenoestrogens in Breast Cancer. S.V. Fernandez and J. Russo. Toxicology Pathology. July 2010; 38(1): 110–122.

Made in the USA
Lexington, KY
22 November 2019

57377541R00203